Building on Early Gains in Afghanistan's Health, Nutrition, and Population Sector

Building on Early Gains in Afghanistan's Health, Nutrition, and Population Sector

Challenges and Options

Tekabe A. Belay,
Editor

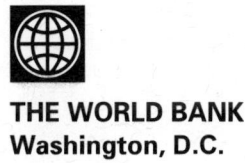

THE WORLD BANK
Washington, D.C.

ISBN: 978-0-8213-8335-3
eISBN: 978-0-8213-8336-0
DOI: 10.1596/978-0-8213-8335-3

Cover image
Bagram, Afghanistan: JACK GUEZ/AFP/Getty Images

Library of Congress Cataloging-in-Publication Data
Building on early gains in Afghanistan's health, nutrition, and population sector : challenges and options / edited by Tekabe A. Belay.
    p. cm.
 Includes bibliographical references and index.
 ISBN 978-0-8213-8335-3 — ISBN 978-0-8213-8336-0 (electronic)
 1. Public health—Afghanistan. 2. Medical care—Afghanistan. 3. Afghanistan—Statistics, Medical. I. Belay, Tekabe A.
 RA541.A3B45 2010
 362.109581—dc22

                                                                              2010013118

Contents

Box

Figures

Tables

Foreword

We are pleased to present this volume, the product of a joint effort of the Ministry of Public Health of the government of Afghanistan, the World Bank, the U.S. Agency for International Development (USAID), and the European Union. The volume provides information on the development of the health system in Afghanistan over the period 2002/03–2007/08 (1381–86 AC), examines the major challenges facing the sector, and provides options for addressing them.

Thanks to the commitment of the government of Afghanistan and the strong leadership of the Ministry of Public Health, and with sustained donor support, the Afghan health sector made significant progress toward achieving the Millennium Development Goals during this period. The number of functioning primary health care facilities more than doubled, coverage of basic health services reached all 34 provinces, the quality of services in publicly financed facilities improved, the infant mortality rate fell 22 percent, and the under-five mortality rate fell 26 percent.

These achievements notwithstanding, significant challenges remain to sustain and further improve the sector performance. This volume aspires to contribute to informed discussions and decision making by all concerned stakeholders.

We would like to express our profound appreciation to the health care professionals working in the field, who often put their lives on the line while providing essential services to the Afghan people. For the dedication of these individuals, the Afghan people and the international community are forever grateful.

Nicholas J. Krafft	William M. Frej	Hansjörg Kretschmer
Country Director	Mission Director	Ambassador to Afghanistan
World Bank	USAID	European Union

Acknowledgments

This volume is a product of a joint effort by the Ministry of Public Health of the government of Afghanistan, the World Bank, the U.S. Agency for International Development (USAID), and the European Union. Such collaborative work is the result of the ongoing partnership between the ministry and its development partners. That partnership was facilitated by the support and guidance of H. E. Dr. S. M. Amin Fatimie, Minister of Public Health, and Dr. Faizullah Kakar, Deputy Minister of Public Health, during the preparation of this book. Their support and guidance are very much appreciated.

This book was produced by Tekabe A. Belay (World Bank). Background papers were prepared by Maryse Dugue (consultant) for the chapter on financing, Goeff King (Liverpool Associates) for the chapter on human resources for health, the GH Tech Group for the chapter on the private sector, Kyhan Natiq (consultant) for the chapter on institutional analysis, and Benjamin Loevinsohn (World Bank) for the chapter on the basic package of health services (BPHS). Valuable inputs from Kees Kostermans are very much appreciated. Comments and suggestions from Kavitha Viswanathan, Ghulam Dastagir Sayed, and Emanuele Capobianco (all from the World Bank) are also acknowledged.

USAID financed the preparation of the background studies for the chapters on human resources for health and participation of the private sector. The European Union funded the assessment of health care finance. Randolph Augustin (USAID, Kabul), Sarah Bernhardt (European Union, Kabul), Timothy Johnston (World Bank), and Agnes Soucat (World Bank) peer reviewed the concept note and the final draft of the original report.

The team would like to thank Julie McLaughlin (Sector Manager, Health, Nutrition, and Population Unit, South Asia Region) for her support and guidance.

Abbreviations

$	All dollar amounts are U.S. dollars unless otherwise indicated.
AC	Afghan calendar
AHS	Afghanistan Household Survey
ARTF	Afghanistan Reconstruction Trust Fund
BCG	Bacillus Calmette-Guerin
BPHS	basic package of health services
CD	compact disk
CDC	Centers for Disease Control
CGHN	Consultative Group on Health and Nutrition
CHA	Coordination of Humanitarian Assistance
CHW	community health worker
DEWS	disease early warning system
DMPA	depot medroxyprogesterone acetate
DPP	Directorate for Provision and Procurement
DPT	diphtheria, pertussis, and tetanus
EPHS	essential package of hospital services
EPI	Expanded Program on Immunization
GAVI	Global Alliance for Vaccines and Immunization
GDA	General Directorate of Administration

GDPP	General Directorate for Policy and Planning
GDPPH	General Directorate of Provincial Public Health
GFATM	Global Fund to Fight AIDS, Tuberculosis and Malaria
HEFD	Health Economics and Finance Department
HMIS	Health Management Information System
HNSS	Health and Nutrition Sector Strategy
IEC/BCC	information, education, and communication/behavior change communication
IMR	infant mortality rate
IUD	intrauterine device
M&E	monitoring and evaluation
MDG	Millennium Development Goal
MICS	Multiple Indicator Cluster Survey
MMR	maternal mortality ratio
MOPH–SM	Ministry of Public Health–Strengthening Mechanism
NGO	nongovernmental organization
NTCC	National Technical Coordination Committee
OPV	oral polio vaccine
PHCC	Provincial Health Coordination Committee
PHO	provincial health office
PPA	performance-based partnership agreement
PPG	performance-based partnership grant
TAG	Technical Advisory Group
UNICEF	United Nations Children's Fund
U5MR	under-five mortality rate
USAID	U.S. Agency for International Development
WHO	World Health Organization

Executive Summary

A number of development partners, including the World Bank, have been actively supporting the health sector in Afghanistan since 2003/04 (1382 AC). Collectively, they invested more than $820 million between 2003 (1382 AC) and 2008/09 (1387 AC) and played key roles in supporting the government in reshaping the country's health sector. This support continues, with all partners starting new projects aimed at further strengthening the sector and building on the successes that have been achieved.

Afghanistan's health system was functioning quite poorly until late 2001 (1380 AC). There was little coverage of preventive and curative health services, for a number of reasons. The prolonged civil war, the shortage of staff in rural areas, and the absence of explicitly articulated national priorities all resulted in limited availability and quality of services. Coverage of services such as skilled birth attendance, antenatal care, and vaccination was very low, with severe consequences for health outcomes. In 2001 (1380 AC), the infant mortality rate (IMR) was estimated at 165 per 1,000 live births, and the under-five mortality rate (U5MR) was estimated at 257 per 1,000 live births. The maternal mortality ratio was as high as 6,507 per 100,000 in some parts of the country.

Afghanistan has made considerable progress since 2001 (1380 AC). A nationwide survey conducted in late 2006 (1385 AC) found that the IMR had fallen 22 percent since 2001 (1380 AC) to 129 per 1,000 live births and the U5MR had fallen 26 percent to 91 per 1,000 live births. Antenatal care coverage increased from less than 5 percent in 2003 (1382 AC) to 32 percent in 2006 (1385 AC), and DTP3 (diphtheria, pertussis, and tetanus vaccine) coverage increased from less than 20 percent to 35 percent. Administrative data indicate that the number of functioning primary health care facilities nearly doubled, from 498 in 2001 (1380 AC) to more than 936 in 2008 (1387 AC). The quality of care in publicly financed facilities also improved. Quality measures increased about 22 percent between 2004 (1383 AC) and 2006 (1385 AC), as assessed by indicators in four different domains based on independent health facility assessments.

The interventions included in the basic package of health services (BPHS) are widely credited as being the major engine behind these successes. The BPHS has been critical in ensuring that all stakeholders working in the health sector in Afghanistan focus on a common strategy established by the Ministry of Public Health (MOPH). The BPHS has therefore also strengthened the stewardship role of the MOPH. The BPHS has established wide "brand recognition," which has made it shorthand for a series of policies and strategies that focus on delivering high-impact primary health care interventions, ensuring that adequate resources and efforts are dedicated to improving coverage of services to the large rural population, improving equity in access to services and maintaining a focus on the poor, and conducting careful monitoring and evaluation (M&E).

Despite this progress, much still remains to be done. Although progress in the health sector is encouraging, it is not sufficient to ensure that Afghanistan will achieve the Millennium Development Goals (MDGs). The U5MR is still 67 percent higher than the average for low-income countries. Similarly, the vaccination coverage rate is still very low by international standards (35 percent versus 65 percent for low-income countries as a whole).

Overcoming the challenges the BPHS faces is critical for its expansion. Although the BPHS has clearly been an important aspect of the success of the health sector in Afghanistan, a number of important challenges remain:

- *Improving coverage and utilization.* The MOPH should build on its experience and continue successful interventions that have increased coverage, including expanding subcenters to reach remote areas; training, deploying, and motivating community health workers; and critically evaluating the various experiments that are being piloted.

- *Enhancing M&E of the BPHS*. M&E is expensive, but it is critical for the success of the BPHS. At a minimum, the MOPH should continue investing in data collection and analysis of data from annual facility surveys and household surveys every two years.
- *Revising the content of the BPHS*. There should be basic principles for revising the content of the BPHS, including, for example, the consistency of the intervention with Afghanistan's health and nutrition sector strategy; the cost-effectiveness of the intervention, taking into account its total cost; the contribution of the intervention to promoting equity; and the feasibility of implementation in the context of Afghanistan.
- *Increasing managerial autonomy*. There is a sense among some stakeholders that the definition of the BPHS is too detailed and that more flexibility should be provided to managers on the ground to adapt the organization of services to local conditions.

Public-private partnerships have proven successful in implementing the BPHS and should continue for the years covered by the next five-year plan (2010–15 [1388–93 AC]). Most health services in Afghanistan are being delivered by nongovernmental organizations (NGOs) under contracts with the MOPH or through grants from a small number of donors. In three provinces near Kabul and parts of rural Kabul province, the MOPH is contracting managers to help strengthen service delivery using MOPH staff. This effort, known as the MOPH Strengthening Mechanism (MOPH–SM), involves the competitive recruitment of managers, the provision of a level of funding similar to that provided to NGOs, and the use of the same M&E mechanisms. Both of these approaches have been considered successful based on facility assessments and administrative data.

External assistance to the sector in support of public-private partnerships grew between 2003 and 2008 (1382–87 AC) and is increasingly "on budget." External assistance increased from less than $100 million in 2003 (1382 AC) to more than $277 million in 2008 (1387 AC). Moreover, the proportion of external finance coming through the budget increased dramatically and will increase further when the United States Agency for International Development (USAID) starts channeling its support through the government.

Despite these gains, the annual rate of increase in funding flowing into the sector has declined, from about 47 percent in 2003/04 (1382 AC) to just 1 percent in 2008/09 (1387 AC). This poses a huge challenge for the MOPH as it aims to expand coverage of the BPHS. The ministry will need to increase its efforts to mobilize resources from diverse sources, including the Afghanistan Reconstruction Trust Fund (ARTF).

Parallel to efforts to increase resources to the sector, the MOPH needs to focus on improving its budget execution. It is hard to argue that the sector needs more resources when it is unable to absorb its current share. Budget execution capacity is low (54 percent), although execution of some off-budget resources is very good. More financial resources could be made available if the ministry improved its administrative and procurement branches in order to increase budget execution.

Increasing resources, by both mobilizing additional funding and improving budget execution, is critical if public resources are to protect the poor from deeper impoverishment from out-of-pocket health care expenses. More than 75 percent of total health care expenditures in Afghanistan are from private sources, almost all of them out-of-pocket payments. About 40 percent of out-of-pocket payments are for medications and supplies, which are purchased mainly from private providers.

In addition to improving budget execution, the MOPH should harness the potential of the private sector to expand services. The private sector provides services to a large segment of the rural population. Recent data show that for first visits, 58 percent of households seek care from private providers. For subsequent visits, the rate goes up to 75 percent. This trend holds across all income groups. The for-profit private sector in rural Afghanistan provides services that complement those provided by the public sector. Although the private sector is the preferred provider for adults, public providers are preferred for maternal and child health services.

Very limited data are available on the quality of services provided by the private sector. The sector is dominated by solo practice physicians, who deliver more than 90 percent of private sector services. The qualifications and quality of care of these solo practice physicians are difficult to regulate or monitor. The only data available to monitor quality are subjective evaluations by patients. According to these evaluations, patients rank private and public providers to be of equal quality, although the data are very difficult to interpret.

The MOPH has a variety of options for enhancing service quality in the private sector. It could encourage private providers to participate in regular quality of care assessments, along the lines of the facility surveys the ministry conducts annually. It could require private providers to participate in health facility surveys or offer incentives to them for doing so.

Large-scale implementation of mandatory participation in quality assessments is not currently viable. Under the mandatory approach, the MOPH would define a minimum acceptable level of quality and assess facilities to ascertain compliance. This approach would be highly demanding in the breadth and depth of information it would require to implement. Enforcing compliance is costly and prone to capture. The current inclination at the MOPH is nevertheless toward using such a regulatory instrument. The ministry should examine its ability to rely exclusively on this instrument. Enforcement capacity, in particular, is a major challenge. The MOPH could use this instrument for licensing, if not for regular monitoring.

The MOPH should explore the use of incentives to improve quality of care by private providers. It could make the accreditation of facilities conditional on attaining a certain performance standard. Private providers could be encouraged to participate in quality assessments to demonstrate their service quality and then be accredited accordingly. The demand for accreditation would increase if the MOPH supplemented the accreditation process by disseminating information on service quality of private providers to the public and selectively contracting with private providers that became accredited.

As important as improving the quality of the private sector is raising the quality of care in the public sector. One impediment to doing so is the lack of qualified health workers, especially in rural areas. The health workforce suffers from three imbalances:

- *Geographic imbalance.* The health care workforce is disproportionately concentrated in cities and periurban areas. Rural areas still suffer from shortages.
- *Gender imbalance.* There is still a shortage of female staff, especially in rural areas.
- *Skills-mix imbalance.* There is still a shortage of staff with public health, reproductive health, and child health skills.

The government should create incentives to make working in the health sector more attractive for women and those willing to work in remote areas. Options include granting preferential admission to medical training for women and those committing to work in remote areas, making postings to preferred locations conditional on first working in a remote area, and making professional development opportunities available in more remote areas.

The MOPH could pilot hiring health facility staff on a contract basis. Doing so would be useful for a number of reasons:

- It would help the MOPH avoid any long-term contingent liabilities that hiring permanent employees would imply.
- It would increase managers' ability to ensure that staff focus on performance.
- It would allow flexible remuneration, which in turn would be a useful instrument for promptly responding to emerging human resource problems.

The MOPH's stewardship role has been central to the success of the BPHS. Before the introduction of the BPHS, NGOs often focused on a variety of priorities. Some emphasized infectious disease control, others reproductive health, and still others noncommunicable disease control. The various NGOs also established different types of facilities and utilized different types of staff. The BPHS has helped ensure that there is a standard national set of priorities and a common overall approach. In particular, it has helped ensure a focus on key health interventions.

The stewardship role of the government is the key to sustaining the gains achieved so far and expanding the BPHS. Although the performance-based partnership agreements and other grants and contracts to NGOs have been successful in delivering the BPHS, they bring the issue of the future role of the MOPH to the forefront. For the ministry to carry out its stewardship role, it needs to have the skilled personnel required to carry out these functions effectively and the organization and institutions that facilitate these functions.

The MOPH needs to strengthen some units and departments that are critical to carrying out its stewardship functions. Doing so will require it to recruit and retain talented Afghans and keep them well motivated. Some stewardship functions were given less priority than others, understandably so at first. However, as the system has grown more complex and the number of stakeholders has increased, the stewardship role of the MOPH has also expanded. Moving forward, the MOPH should establish or strengthen the units required to take on more stewardship functions and attract staff with the needed skills and motivation. These units include a unit to work with the private sector and a unit for health care financing responsible for mobilizing resources and tracking expenditures.

The ministry should build on its experience in hiring skilled and motivated staff on a competitive basis. The MOPH is among the few ministries that are seen as successful in expanding services throughout the country through its partnership with NGOs. Such partnerships would not have been possible had the ministry not been able to manage and guide the operations of the NGOs. Such management and guidance have been partly credited to the skills and motivation of the staff hired on a competitive basis and paid market salaries.

In addition to strengthening units and departments in Kabul, the MOPH should use the immense potential of its provincial offices to broaden its stewardship role. The Provincial Health Offices (PHOs) should be strengthened to play a key role in supervising the performance of NGOs and providing technical guidance. They should also be strengthened to work effectively with the for-profit private sector, so that regulatory functions are gradually transferred to the PHOs.

Introduction

Afghanistan's health sector has come a long way since 2002 (1381 AC). A number of development partners, especially the World Bank, the European Union, and the U.S. Agency for International Development (USAID), have been key supporters of the government of Afghanistan's effort to rebuild and strengthen the health sector. Together the three donors invested more than $820 million between 2003/04 and 2008/09 (1382–87 AC) and played key roles in helping the government reshape the health sector. This support continues, with all partners starting new projects aimed at further strengthening the sector and building on the successes that have been achieved.

This book is a collaborative effort by the Ministry of Public Health (MOPH), the World Bank, the European Union, and USAID. Its purpose is to document the achievements made so far, identify areas that need to be strengthened, and present policy options to help guide the government and its development partners on the way forward.

Objectives

The book aims to document the achievements in rebuilding Afghanistan's health system over the period 2002–08 (1381–87 AC); contribute to the development of a set of practical policy options that will further increase

1

the quality, availability, and use of health services by the poor and other vulnerable groups; provide policy options for the MOPH as it defines its future role in the sector; and suggest how the development partners can best support the efforts of the government. It focuses on practical issues and examines a number of policies that are feasible to implement.

Scope and Methodology

The topics covered were identified after extensive consultation with the MOPH and its development partners. These topics were identified as the most pressing and as areas in which synthesized documentation is needed.

As part of this volume, four studies were undertaken to fill gaps in knowledge:

- A survey was conducted to describe the structure of the private health sector in rural Afghanistan.
- An overview of health care financing was produced to provide a picture of the resource envelope available for the sector, as well as the sources and uses of funds.
- An assessment was completed to provide an overview of human resources for health, including the size, distribution, and skill mix of the health workforce.
- An analysis was carried out to assess the institutional capacity of the ministry to carry out its stewardship functions effectively.

Structure and Outline of the Book

The book is organized as follows. Chapters 1–4 tell a coherent story about the achievements of the sector between 2002 and 2008 (1381–87 AC), the financial resources used to achieve the results, and the contribution the private sector has made to the achievements. Chapters 5–8 look forward. They identify the challenges the sector is facing in meeting human resource needs, expanding the coverage of the basic package of health services (BPHS), and increasing the institutional capacity of the MOPH. Chapter 8 summarizes the lessons learned and provides options for moving forward.

Chapter 1 presents the health sector in the context of Afghanistan's overall economic growth and efforts to reduce poverty. It describes the national health and nutrition sector strategy and the development of the health system since 2001 (1380 AC).

Chapter 2 discusses the development of Afghanistan's health system and its performance since 2001 (1380 AC). It describes the changes in health outcomes, particularly in child mortality rates and maternal mortality ratios; progress in the coverage of health promotion, preventive and curative services, and utilization rates and patterns; and examines the quality of care based on the health facility assessments.

Chapter 3 assesses the sources and uses of financial resource flows into the sector. It also examines the budget process and structure and issues around donor funding.

Chapter 4 looks at the emerging for-profit private sector in rural Afghanistan. It describes its current structure, reviews the services and quality of care it provides, and explores options the MOPH faces in ensuring that the sector contributes to meeting national health objectives.

Chapter 5 addresses human resources for health. It describes the mix and distribution of human resources and focuses on three issues the sector is facing: geographic imbalance, gender imbalance, and skills-mix imbalance.

Chapter 6 focuses on improving the coverage of primary health care by strengthening the delivery of the BPHS. It summarizes the evidence on structural interventions, such as the introduction of subcenters and community health workers; discusses issues surrounding revision of the BPHS; and examines monitoring and evaluation to track the performance of the primary health care sector.

Chapter 7 assesses the institutional capacity of the ministry to carry out its stewardship functions. It examines the government's stewardship role and its future role in health service delivery. The chapter aims to answer two broad questions: Does the ministry have the right institutions and necessary skills to carry out its functions? To what extent is it carrying out its functions?

Chapter 8 presents concluding remarks and summarizes lessons for the way forward.

CHAPTER 1

Background

This chapter presents the country context within which the health sector operates. It describes the economic, social, and security situation in Afghanistan within which policies affecting the health sector should be framed.

Health, Macroeconomic Environment, and Poverty

The performance of Afghanistan's economy between 2002/03–2007/08 (1381–86 AC) was strong. Between 2002/03 and 2006/07 (1381–85 AC), real GDP growth averaged 15 percent a year, and inflation was brought down to single-digit levels in 2006/07 (1385 AC). Revenue collection also improved significantly, rising from 4.7 percent of GDP in 2003/04 (1382 AC) to 7 percent in 2007/08 (1385 AC).

The performance of the health sector in Afghanistan appears to be in line with the country's observed economic growth. It is well documented that investment in health contributes to sustained economic growth and stability. At the macro level, health endowments and investments in health are found to be sound predictors of economic growth (Stiglitz 2002). At the micro level, differences in health status explain differences in output per worker almost as well as differences in physical capital (Weil 2001). Economic growth, in turn, is one of the most important drivers of health system performance and health outcomes.

Poverty and Health

Poverty is widespread in Afghanistan, especially in rural areas. Estimates from the National Risk and Vulnerability Assessment (World Bank 2005) show that 30 percent of the population of Afghanistan lives below the poverty line. Poverty is exacerbated by the health shocks individual households experience. Health shocks are the most important events that drive rural Afghan households into poverty, and the frequency and magnitude of such shocks are large among poor households (World Bank 2005). Hence, providing effective health services helps reduce poverty.

Poverty in Afghanistan correlates strongly with both household health and demographic characteristics. The health status and dependency ratio of a household affects its labor supply and earnings. Having a large number of children makes poor households more vulnerable to the lack of maternal and child health services.

The Health and Nutrition Sector Strategy

One of the pillars of the Afghanistan national development strategy (2008–13 [1387–91 AC]) is economic and social development. The strategy's main objectives are reducing poverty, ensuring sustainable economic development through a private sector–led market economy, improving human development indicators, and making significant progress toward meeting the Millennium Development Goals.

The national health and nutrition sector strategy (2008–13 [1387–91 AC]) elaborates on the national development strategy. It sets four ambitious targets to be attained by the end of 2013 (1391 AC):

- Reduce the maternal mortality ratio by 50 percent from the 2000 (1379 AC) level.
- Reduce infant and under-five mortality rates by 50 percent from the 2000 (1379 AC) level.
- Increase physical access to the basic package of health services (BPHS) by increasing the proportion of people living within two hours' walking distance of a health facility from the 2008/09 (1387 AC) level of 65–90 percent.
- Attain full immunization coverage.

The health and nutrition sector strategy presents nine core programs related to health care services and five related to institutional development that are instrumental to attaining these targets.

Security

Afghanistan still faces serious security challenges. Terrorism, foreign interference, and instability and weak capacity in governance are preventing the government from establishing effective control in some regions of the country, particularly in the south and southeast. Land mines and unexploded ordnance remain significant threats, with some 5,000 civilians killed or wounded in mine explosions since 2001 (1380 AC). Only 2 of the country's 34 provinces are completely clear of mines, and only part of the country is accessible. The United Nations Department of Safety and Security (UNDSS) rates the entire eastern, southern, and southeastern regions of Afghanistan as "volatile" and not accessible by Bank staff. Within provinces considered secure, some districts are not accessible for security reasons.

The precarious security situation poses a risk to all development activities, particularly health service delivery, which involves working in rural areas and requires considerable movement (delivering drugs, conducting outreach activities, providing supervision). The provision of services in insecure areas is one of the biggest challenges. In Helmand province, for instance, 40 percent of health facilities have been closed because of insecurity, six facilities have been destroyed, and health workers have been killed. It is a challenge posting and retaining female health workers in insecure areas, and they are critical for maternal health services.

The results of insecurity are evident in the utilization of health services. Insecurity in parts of the country appears to be having a significant effect on the ability of the Ministry of Public Health (MOPH) and its partners to deliver the BPHS, as well as on the ability of patients to access services. The work of an Afghan nongovernmental organization (NGO) working in both a secure (Saripul) and an insecure (Helmand) province demonstrates the effect of security on utilization: although the two provinces started at roughly similar levels of health facility utilization, improvements have been much more rapid in Saripul.

The government has adopted various ways to increase utilization of health services despite the difficult security situation. The key elements of these activities include the following:

- Conditional cash transfer schemes for well-child visits and birth deliveries in a facility

- A performance-based incentive scheme for community health workers
- A security allowance for skilled health workers on top of the national salary policy, to keep insecure facilities appropriately staffed
- Establishment of subcenters on a pilot basis
- Establishment of a monitoring system by the provincial health office and members of the community.

Evolution of the Health System

Afghanistan's health system has evolved as the roles of the government and NGOs have changed. The last years of the Taliban, for instance, saw NGOs playing the major role in health services provision, with little coordination or guidance from the ministry. The government is now a major player. The MOPH leads the sector by formulating policies and coordinating the efforts of various stakeholders.

Organization of the Public Health Service Delivery System

The pyramidal structure of Afghanistan's health delivery system is similar to that observed in other developing countries. It is structured as follows:

- Health posts are intended to be the first point of contact for health care services. These posts are staffed with male and female community health workers who are not health professionals but who have received targeted training. Each facility covers a population of 1,000–1,900.
- Subcenters came into effect as a result of innovations to reach remote and geographically difficult areas. A typical facility is staffed with a male nurse and a community midwife and covers a population of 2,000–15,000.
- Basic health centers provide outpatient services and supervise subcenters and health posts. A typical center is staffed with a nurse, a community midwife, and two vaccinators. Each basic health center covers a population of 15,000–30,000.
- Comprehensive health centers provide limited inpatient services. They are staffed with male and female doctors, male and female midwives, and laboratory and pharmacy technicians. Each center covers a population of 30,000–100,000.
- District hospitals serve as referral points at the district level. Each is staffed with obstetricians/gynecologists, a surgeon, an anesthetist, a pediatrician, midwives, laboratory and X-ray technicians, a pharmacist, and a dentist and dental technician. Each district hospital covers a population of 100,000–300,000.

- Provincial hospitals serve as referral points at the provincial level.
- Regional hospitals serve as referral points for groups of provinces.
- National hospitals and tertiary care hospitals are located mainly in Kabul.

Role of the Private Sector
In addition to public facilities, there exists a largely unregulated private sector, which operates mainly at the basic care level. The private sector provides a limited scope of services compared with those offered by the public sector and NGOs. This part of the health delivery system is used frequently, particularly by poorer households, however. It has the potential to considerably improve access to essential services, as is discussed in chapter 4.

Role of NGOs
Before 2001 (1380 AC), health services in Afghanistan were provided by NGOs, with little coordination or guidance from the ministry. During the period of Taliban control, fewer restrictions were imposed on the health sector than on other social sectors. As a result, significant external assistance continued, with externally funded NGOs playing a dominant role.

When the Taliban were removed from power in late 2001 (1380 AC), 80 percent of the health facilities in the country were managed or supported by NGOs. There was little coordination of activities, there was no standard package of services, and the government had very little influence over the activities of NGOs. Health facilities were situated primarily in accessible urban or more secure rural areas, leaving large parts of the population unserved. In addition, NGO activities focused on individual facilities rather than clearly defined populations or geographic areas, resulting in an irrational distribution of services, with a patchwork of NGO clinics with obvious duplication and inefficiencies. There was a lack of services in remote rural areas and no accountability of NGOs for tangible results.

Development of Packages of Health Services
In response to the fragmentation and lack of coordination of efforts of the various agents operating before 2002 (1381 AC), the MOPH made the development of a standard package of health services its main priority. It developed the BPHS and the essential package of hospital services (EPHS) in 2002 (1381 AC), in collaboration with its partners.

The BPHS includes a set of high-impact interventions aimed at addressing the principal health problems of the population, with an emphasis on the health of women and children, the two most vulnerable groups. In developing the BPHS, the MOPH sought to provide a standardized package of basic services that would form the core of service delivery for all primary care facilities and promote the redistribution of health services by providing equitable access, especially in underserved areas.

The EPHS identifies a standardized package of hospital services for each level of hospital. It provides guidance on how the hospital sector should be staffed, equipped, and provided with materials and pharmaceuticals and promotes a referral system that integrates the BPHS with hospitals.

Since the beginning of 2004 (1382 AC), the MOPH has been able to assert its stewardship over the health sector by developing the BPHS and partnering with NGOs to implement it. With support from donor funding, it has contracted with NGOs for the delivery of the BPHS. This partnership has been essential, as NGOs were already running most facilities in 2001 (1380 AC) and are experienced with the challenges of delivering services in Afghanistan. The MOPH has used contracts with NGOs to ensure that all providers are implementing the BPHS in accordance with its technical guidelines and that all providers are clearly responsible and held accountable for defined geographical areas and populations.

Initially, the MOPH, NGOs, and development partners all had concerns about the feasibility of contracting out health service provision in a country in which the private sector is sometimes viewed as excessively profit oriented and the sense of centralization is strong. At the same time, the NGOs were hesitant to give up the relative independence they had enjoyed for years.

Partly because of these concerns, the MOPH participates in delivering services in three small provinces near Kabul (Kapisa, Panjshir, and Parwan), with management contracted in. This approach is known as the MOPH Strengthening Mechanism (MOPH–SM). MOPH staff in these three provinces receive salaries comparable to those provided by NGOs (and in keeping with the national salary policy). Financial resources are channeled through the provincial governments, with financial management support provided by local consultants. In addition, NGOs have been contracted to train some service providers, including community midwives and community health workers.

By 2008/09 (1387 AC), NGOs were delivering the BPHS in 31 of Afghanistan's 34 provinces, with financial support from donors. Support is provided by the United States Agency for International Development (USAID) (13 provinces), the World Bank (11 provinces), and the European Commission (10 provinces). Three of the 11 provinces supported by the Bank are following the MOPH–SM model.

As of 2008/09 (1387 AC), about 77 percent of Afghanistan's population had access to basic services. The quality of care is independently measured on a regular basis, with results made widely available.

Contracting Arrangements

Contracting with NGOs has worked well in Afghanistan and proven to be a way for the government to rapidly regain and maintain policy leadership. By setting priorities, allocating geographical responsibility, providing financing, and carefully monitoring performance, the MOPH has been able to provide direction to what was previously an uncoordinated and chaotic system. Serious constraints, such as scarce human resources, lack of physical facilities, and logistical challenges, have been addressed by giving NGOs a fair degree of autonomy but holding them accountable for achieving national priorities.

The MOPH has contracted with NGOs on a large scale. About a quarter of the contracts (27 percent) are with international NGOs. As of 2008/09 (1387 AC), 82 percent of the population lived in districts in which primary care services were provided by NGOs under contracts with the MOPH or through grants to the NGOs (largely from the three donors).

There are some differences depending on the source of financing, but there are important commonalities, and the approaches appear to be getting more consistent over time. All grants and contracts are based on the delivery of the BPHS, as defined by the MOPH. All of the approaches do the following:

- Assign clear geographical responsibility to the NGOs (typically for entire provinces, with populations of about 150,000–1 million).
- Employ competitive selection of NGOs.
- Promote convergence toward common indicators of success.
- Invoke a credible threat of sanctions if an NGO does not perform well (one international NGO had its contract terminated).

Contracting arrangements vary slightly among the three major donors and are managed largely by the MOPH (table 1.1). The European Union (EU) office in Kabul manages contracts financed by the EU. The Health Economics and Finance Department (HEFD) (previously the Grants and Contracts Management Unit [GCMU]) of the MOPH manages contracts financed by the World Bank and USAID. The role of

Table 1.1 MOPH Contracting Schemes with USAID, the World Bank, and the European Union

Donor	Number of provinces covered	Flow of funds	Contract management	Performance-based elements	Monitoring and evaluation
U.S. Agency for International Development	13	Previously through a third party, currently from USAID to MOPH	Health Economics and Finance Department	No bonus, but extension of contract is conditional on good performance	Small-scale household surveys
World Bank	11 (8 contracted with NGOs, 3 contracted with MOPH–SM)	From Ministry of Finance to MOPH	Health Economics and Finance Department	Monetary bonus of up to 10 percent of the contract value provided: 1 percent every six months during the life of the project for a 10 percentage point increase over the baseline in the Balanced Score Card, 5 percent at end of the project for a 50 percentage point increase	Annual facility survey and household survey conducted by third party covering the entire country; quarterly reports
European Union	10	From European Union to NGOs	European Union	None	Third-party evaluation in EU provinces; annual report to European Union, quarterly reports to MOPH

Source: Waldman, Strong, and Wali 2006.
Note: EU = European Union; MOPH = Ministry of Public Health; MOPH–SM = Ministry of Public Health–Strengthening Mechanism; NGO = nongovernmental organization; USAID = U.S. Agency for International Development.

HEFD was envisioned as one of coordination and oversight of NGOs implementing the BPHS throughout the country. In addition to these original functions, the HEFD is now carrying out a number of additional activities, including providing technical assistance and management support to several line departments of the MOPH, coordinating donors, and responding to urgent policy-related requests from the minister and deputy ministers.

The MOPH monitors the implementation of the BPHS through its central departments, including the HEFD. The MOPH monitors service delivery through the Health Management Information System (HMIS) and through facility and community surveys carried out by a third party. The HEFD handles the fiduciary aspects of implementing the BPHS, including financial management, procurement, disbursement, and audit functions.

Evidence for Future Directions

Global experience suggests that NGOs perform better than ministries of public health in delivering direct health services. Although critics of contracting arrangements argue that the government should be responsible for service delivery, accumulating evidence from other countries suggests that contracting with NGOs may provide better results than direct government provision of the same services.

In a recent review of global experience, 10 evaluated examples of contracting were analyzed. All 10 concluded that contracting is very effective and that improvements can be rapid (Loevinsohn and Harding 2004). Four of the 10 cases included controlled before and after evaluations. These evaluations demonstrated an impact of 3–26 percentage points on important indicators of performance (as measured by the median double difference: follow-up minus baseline in the experimental group minus follow-up minus baseline in the control). Six of the 10 studies compared contractor performance with government provision of the same services; all six found that contractors were more effective than the government in providing services. NGOs performed better even when they had fewer resources than public institutions.

Evidence from Afghanistan shows that the MOPH–SM performs better than traditional provision of direct service by the MOPH. Based on before and after data, analysis of the performance of the two methods finds that service quality in MOPH–SM facilities improved significantly compared with MOPH facilities (Belay 2009). The quality indicators include functionality of equipment, availability of drugs, laboratory functionality, provider knowledge, and adherence to clinical guidelines. The analysis also shows that MOPH–SM facilities have done a better job of attracting female patients than MOPH facilities and that health worker satisfaction is much higher in MOPH–SM facilities.

The evidence on the relative performance of contracting with NGOs and using the MOPH–SM is not as strong in Afghanistan as it is in other countries. The data show that overall performance is comparable but that contracted NGOs perform slightly better on service coverage. In terms of quality of care, there is no significant difference between MOPH–SM facilities and contracted NGOs. Patients express an equal level of satisfaction with services in both settings, but contracted NGOs are more pro-poor than MOPH–SM facilities.

The potential gains from expanding the MOPH–SM to the hospital sector are enormous. Although it is premature to conclude that the MOPH–SM provides better service than NGOs, it is clear that it has out-performed the traditional government health service delivery model. The success of the MOPH–SM experiment in BPHS delivery could be replicated in the implementation of the EPHS, where the traditional form of management prevails. However, such intervention should be made cautiously, as the hospital sector is more complex and more prone to the influence of powerful groups with vested interests than is the primary care sector. Moreover, the capacity of the MOPH–SM needs to be strengthened before it can manage hospitals on a larger scale. Small-scale piloting of the MOPH–SM is suggested to mobilize buy-in from stakeholders and gradually build capacity in hospital management.

The MOPH–SM is a unique arrangement that signifies a departure from traditional government health service delivery. Three features of the approach stand out as contributing to its success and should be kept in mind if the model is scaled up:

- The MOPH–SM partners with NGOs in a number of areas, including the education of community midwives and health workers and the management of hospitals.
- Managers of facilities have broader authority to retain or fire staff than is usual in publicly managed facilities. Although it is extremely difficult to fire a civil servant, most of the MOPH–SM staff were upgraded to a higher salary scale through the Priority Reform Restructuring

program, which allowed managers to retain or demote them to the regular salary scale.

- Service delivery by NGOs in non–MOPH–SM provinces created an implicit benchmark against which the performance of the MOPH–SM is measured. Moreover, NGOs are providing health services at comparable costs, which presents a competitive environment for the MOPH–SM.

CHAPTER 2

Health Status and Performance of the Sector

Although progress since 2003 (1382 AC) has been substantial, Afghanistan continues to have some of the poorest health indicators in the world. The key challenges the country faces include high infant and under-five mortality rates; a very high maternal mortality ratio, with most deaths preventable if more births were attended by skilled providers and properly referred; poor sanitation and malnutrition; and a high burden of disease from malaria and tuberculosis. This chapter describes progress made in these key areas and identifies some of the impediments to improving the health status of the population of Afghanistan.

Health Outcomes

Child health, maternal health, and nutritional status are poor in Afghanistan, although child mortality rates have declined sharply in recent years. Lack of adequate nutrition contributes to both child and maternal mortality.

Child Health

Afghanistan has some of the highest infant and under-five mortality rates in the world, although both rates have steadily declined since

1960 (1339 AC) (figures 2.1 and 2.2). In 2002 (1381 AC) the number of deaths per 1,000 live births was estimated at 165 for infants and 257 for children under five (UNICEF 2004). Considerable investment in the health sector since 2003 (1382 AC) has contributed to reductions in both mortality rates: the under-five mortality rate dropped 26 percent (from 257 to 191) and the infant mortality rate dropped 22 percent (from 165 to 129) between 2003 (1382 AC) and 2006 (1385 AC).

The Millennium Development Goal (MDG) target for Afghanistan is to reduce the infant mortality rate to 82 per 1,000 live births and the under-five mortality rate to 128 deaths per 1,000 live births by 2015 (1394 AC). If these targets are to be achieved, Afghanistan needs to register progress at a higher rate than it did between 2003 (1382 AC) and 2006 (1385 AC).

Figure 2.1   Trends in Infant Mortality Rate in Afghanistan, South Asia, and Sub-Saharan Africa, 1960–2006 (1339–85 AC)

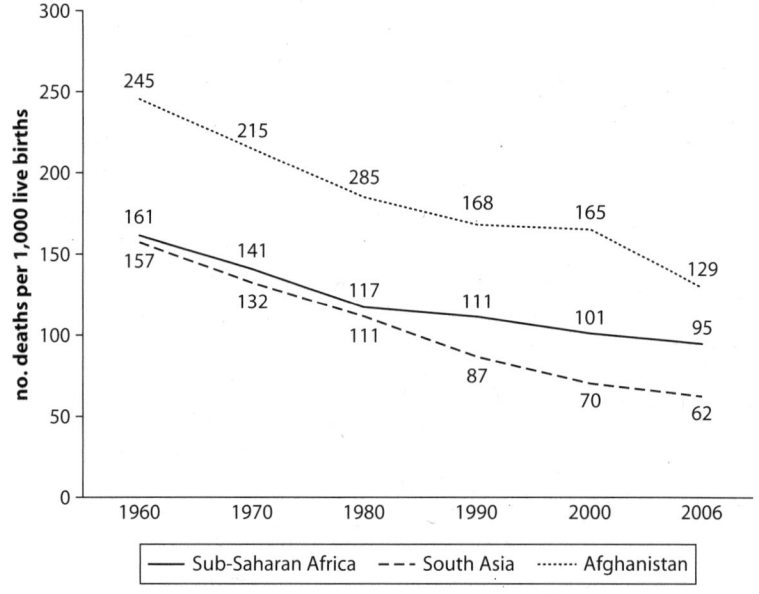

Sources: For Afghanistan: UNICEF 2004; Johns Hopkins Bloomberg School of Public Health and Indian Institute of Health Management Research 2007; Ministry of Public Health 2008c. For South Asia and Sub-Saharan Africa: UNICEF and others 2007.

Figure 2.2   Trends in Under-Five Mortality Rate in Afghanistan, South Asia, and Sub-Saharan Africa, 1960–2006 (1339–85 AC)

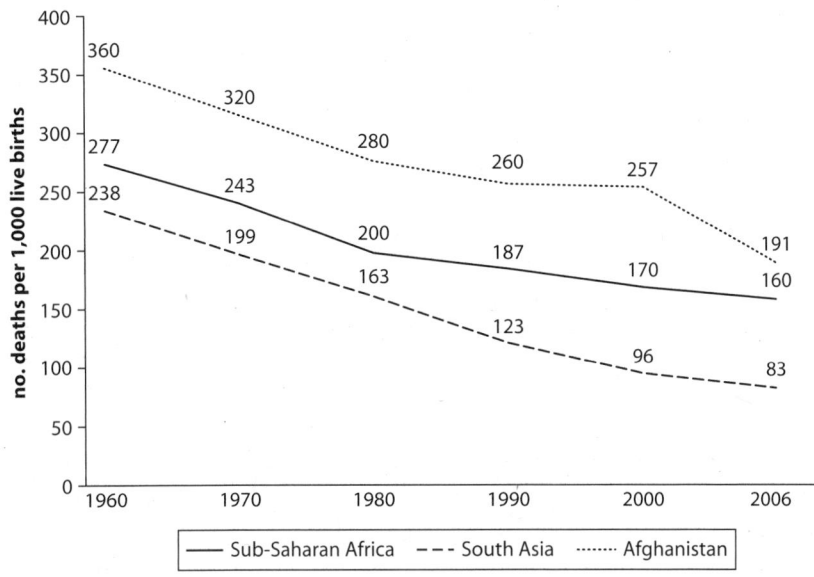

Sources: For Afghanistan: UNICEF 2007; Johns Hopkins Bloomberg School of Public Health and Indian Institute of Health Management Research 2007; Ministry of Public Health 2008c. For South Asia and Sub-Saharan Africa: UNICEF and others 2007.

Maternal Health

The maternal mortality ratio is extremely high in Afghanistan: the most recent data show 1,800 maternal deaths per 100,000 live births (WHO 2007). These model-based estimates are similar to estimates produced in an earlier study by the United Nations Children's Fund (UNICEF) and the Centers for Disease Control (CDC) in four districts in Afghanistan, which found a maternal mortality ratio of 1,600 (Bartlett and others 2005). The last maternal mortality survey was conducted in 2002 (1381 AC). Given the expansion of maternal and child health services, more recent estimates from an upcoming Ministry of Public Health (MOPH) survey are expected to show improvements.

Nutrition and Micronutrients

The nutritional status of Afghans is poor. Many of the recent nutrition data come from an MOPH/Tufts/CDC national nutrition survey of 900 children conducted in 2004 (MOPH and others 2004). This survey included anthropometric measures of children 6–59 months and of women of childbearing age (14–49 years). The results indicate that among children under five, the prevalence of stunting is "very high" (54 percent), the prevalence of underweight is "high" (40 percent), and the prevalence of wasting is "medium" (7 percent), according to World Health Organization (WHO) classifications. Thirty-seven percent of Afghan children are already stunted by 12 months. The prevalence of underweight and wasting increases in children older than 6 months of age, with the highest rates seen among children 6–24 months.

Lack of basic health services is partly responsible for the poor nutritional outcomes, which in turn contribute to high infant and child mortality rates. For instance, severe diarrhea can lead to acute malnutrition, and repeated episodes of diarrhea during infancy and childhood can stunt growth. The prevalence of diarrhea in the two weeks before the survey was conducted was 46 percent among children 6–59 months (MOPH and others 2004). It has fallen markedly since then: according to the 2006 (1385 AC) Afghanistan Household Survey, the estimate of diarrhea among children in that age category was about 18 percent (Ministry of Public Health 2006).

Nutritional status is also a key factor in reducing maternal and neonatal mortality. Improvements in maternal and child health go hand in hand with improvements in nutritional status. Iron-deficiency anemia in pregnant women, for example, can increase the risk of poor pregnancy outcomes. It is alarming, therefore, that 48 percent of nonpregnant women of reproductive age were classified as iron deficient (MOPH and others 2004). Almost 75 percent of nonpregnant women had very low urinary iodine levels. Iodine deficiency can increase the risk of pregnancy complications, stillbirths, neonatal mortality, and growth retardation.

Performance of the Health Care System

Overall utilization of health care services has increased significantly in Afghanistan, albeit not uniformly across the country. Utilization is positively correlated with wealth status.

Trends in Key Health Service Delivery Indicators

Although health care utilization remains low, it has increased continuously in recent years. The annual number of per capita outpatient department visits increased from 0.60 in 2006 (1385 AC) to 1.04 in 2008 (1387 AC), according to the Health Management Information System (HMIS). Increased utilization of outpatient services, together with increased coverage of key maternal and child health services and improvements in quality of care, indicates that the perceived and real value of health care services is increasing. Not everyone is benefiting equally from these gains, however. The poor and populations in remote areas are less likely to use services than the wealthier and people in less remote areas. Although progress has been made in reducing inequality, much more remains to be done.

Child health services. Positive developments in immunization coverage have contributed to the decline in under-five mortality. Vaccinations for BCG (Bacillus Calmette-Guerin); polio; and DPT (diphtheria, pertussis, and tetanus) increased significantly between 2003 (1382 AC) and 2006 (1385 AC), although measles immunization and vitamin A coverage dropped (table 2.1). Some immunizations are given through campaigns (polio and measles vaccinations are given together with vitamin A supplementation, for example), so coverage depends on the frequency of campaigns. Polio vaccination levels increased as a result of frequent polio campaigns as part of the global polio eradication efforts. Measles vaccination coverage dropped between 2003 (1382 AC) and 2006 (1385 AC) because a large campaign was undertaken in 2003 (1382 AC) but not repeated before the survey was undertaken in 2006 (1385 AC).

Reproductive health services. Coverage of reproductive health services increased significantly between 2003 (1382 AC) and 2006 (1385 AC) (table 2.2). Use of contraceptives, skilled antenatal care, and skilled birth attendants all increased by a factor of at least three over the period.

Table 2.1   Coverage of Immunization and Vitamin A Supplementation, 2003–06 (1382–85 AC)

(percentage of children 12–23 months)

Immunization/supplementation	2003 Multiple Indicator Cluster Survey (median estimate)	2005 National Risk and Vulnerability Assessment (mean estimate)	2006 Afghanistan Household Survey (mean estimate)
Bacillus Calmette-Guerin (BCG)	56.5	58.8	70.2
Oral polio vaccine (OPV3)	29.9	49.2	69.7
Diphtheria, pertussis, and tetanus (DPT3)	19.5	16.7	34.6
Measles	75.6	52.8	62.6
Full immunization	15.5	11.2	27.1
Vitamin A	90.3	44.8	79.5

Sources: UNICEF 2004; Afghanistan Household Survey (Ministry of Public Health 2006).

Table 2.2   Trends in Coverage of Key Reproductive Health Services, 2003–06 (1382–85 AC)

Indicator	2003 Multiple Indicator Cluster Survey (median estimate)	2005 National Risk and Vulnerability Assessment (mean estimate)	2006 Afghanistan Household Survey (mean estimate)
Contraceptive prevalence rate	5.1	10.4	15.4
Skilled antenatal care	4.6	12.6	32.3
Skilled birth attendant	6.0	8.4	18.9

Sources: UNICEF 2004; Afghanistan Household Survey (Ministry of Public Health 2006).
Note: Contraceptive prevalence rate = proportion of currently married women 10–49 using modern contraceptive. Skilled antenatal care = proportion of women 10–49 attended by skilled health care professional at least once during pregnancy in past two years. Skilled birth attendant = proportion of women 10–49 attended by skilled professional during childbirth in past two years.

Antenatal care coverage increased the most, rising from 4.6 percent to 32.3 percent.

Equity in Health Service Utilization

Wealth status is the strongest predictor of care-seeking behavior in Afghanistan. A multivariate analysis using a 2004 (1383 AC) household survey conducted in the catchment areas of the health facilities shows that people from households in the wealthiest quintile are twice as likely to seek care as people from the poorest quintile.

Care seeking is also related to the type of illness. People experiencing diarrhea or intestinal problems are 30–40 percent more likely to seek care than those with respiratory problems, fever, or other conditions. Age, gender, head of household status, and the interaction terms of wealth and education and gender and age are not significant as determinants of health care–seeking behavior (Steinhardt and others 2009).

Child health services. Immunization rates vary significantly by wealth status (table 2.3). Children from the poorest households are almost twice as likely as children from the wealthiest households to have received no vaccinations. This difference is less stark for OPV3, which is delivered by campaign-based vaccination.

Reproductive health services. Wealth status also affects the use of reproductive health services in Afghanistan. Prevalence rates for contraceptives, use of antenatal care, and share of births attended by a skilled

Table 2.3   Immunization Coverage, by Wealth Quintile
(percentage of children 12–23 months)

Wealth quintile	BCG	OPV3	DPT1	DPT2	DPT3	Measles	All vaccinations	No vaccinations
Lowest (poorest)	52.9	63.0	44.5	35.1	21.5	48.5	14.3	20.9
Second	67.5	63.7	57.7	45.4	32.6	59.9	23.0	14.1
Middle	74.6	68.7	59.5	47.7	35.6	64.6	28.1	13.1
Fourth	78.0	76.6	68.2	57.6	39.0	68.5	31.1	10.1
Highest (richest)	81.0	77.7	73.8	59.4	45.2	73.3	39.9	11.3
Overall	70.2	69.7	60.4	48.7	34.6	62.6	27.1	14.1

Source: Afghanistan Household Survey (Ministry of Public Health 2006).
Note: BCG = Bacillus Calmette-Guerin; DPT = diphtheria, pertussis, and tetanus; OPV = oral polio vaccine.

attendant and taking place in an institution are all much higher for women from the wealthiest households.

Couples in households from the wealthiest quintile are more likely than other couples to use contraceptives (table 2.4). Nationally, 15.5 percent of currently married women are using at least one method of modern contraception; women from households in the wealthiest quintile are almost four times as likely to use contraception as women from households in the poorest quintile.

Use of antenatal care is also related to wealth (table 2.5). Women from households in the highest wealth quintile are more than twice as likely to use skilled antenatal care as women from households in the poorest quintile. They are about twice as likely to use a midwife for antenatal care (10.9 percent versus 21.8 percent) and almost four times as likely to use a physician (5.9 percent versus 22.8 percent). The smaller wealth gap in the use of midwives may indicate a combination of preferences and physical access.

Overall, levels of use of skilled attendants are low, with just 19 percent of women attended by a skilled birth attendant. The difference between the poor and the wealthier is greater for the use of skilled birth attendants than for antenatal care or contraceptive usage (table 2.6). Women from the wealthiest quintile are more than six times as likely as women from the poorest quintile to be attended by a physician while giving birth and almost five times as likely to use a midwife. The use of unskilled providers is higher among women from poorer households.

It is still rare for deliveries to take place in an institution in Afghanistan: more than 85 percent of births take place at home. Women from the

Table 2.4   Use of Modern Contraception, by Wealth Quintile
(percentage of currently married women 10–49 years of age)

Wealth quintile	Use at least one modern method	Method used				
		Pill	*DMPA*	*Condom*	*IUD*	*Female sterilization*
Lowest (poorest)	7.4	3.4	3.2	0.5	0.4	0.2
Second	13.0	7.6	3.8	1.8	0.2	0.4
Middle	13.4	6.4	4.8	1.8	0.6	1.1
Fourth	19.1	10.5	6.7	3.4	1.6	0.5
Highest (richest)	27.8	14.4	9.1	4.0	2.7	1.6
Overall	15.5	8.1	5.4	2.2	1.0	0.7

Source: Afghanistan Household Survey (Ministry of Public Health 2006).
Note: DMPA = depot medroxyprogesterone acetate (Depo-Provera®); IUD = intrauterine device.

Table 2.5   Use of Skilled Antenatal Care, by Wealth Quintile
(percentage of currently married women who delivered in past two years)

Wealth quintile	Receives any skilled antenatal care	Care provider used			
		Physician	*Midwife*	*Nurse*	*Community health worker*
Lowest (poorest)	18.6	5.9	10.9	0.0	1.8
Second	26.2	10.0	13.7	0.2	2.3
Middle	37.2	16.2	18.4	0.5	2.2
Fourth	36.8	17.2	16.5	0.9	2.1
Highest (richest)	47.9	22.8	21.8	0.2	3.1
Overall	32.3	13.7	15.9	0.3	2.3

Source: Afghanistan Household Survey (Ministry of Public Health 2006).

Table 2.6   Use of Skilled Providers for Delivery, by Wealth Quintile
(percentage of currently married women who delivered in past two years)

Wealth quintile	Use of skilled birth attendant	Skilled provider		Unskilled provider		
		Physician	*Midwife*	*Traditional birth attendant*	*Relative or friend*	*No provider*
Lowest (poorest)	7.3	2.6	4.7	18.2	67.4	6.1
Second	11.6	3.1	8.6	25.7	49.0	5.9
Middle	19.0	6.8	12.2	26.2	43.5	3.1
Fourth	22.9	10.1	12.8	18.2	50.7	4.7
Highest (richest)	38.4	16.1	22.3	12.8	40.4	1.9
Overall	19.0	7.3	11.6	20.4	53.8	4.5

Source: Afghanistan Household Survey (Ministry of Public Health 2006).

wealthiest quintile are 10 times as likely as women from the poorest quintile to deliver in a facility (table 2.7). Among deliveries that take place in institutions, hospitals are the most common setting. The rich-poor gap is highest in hospitals, with 24.1 percent of the wealthiest women and only 2.2 percent of the poorest women giving birth in hospitals. There is a clear need to improve access to and utilization of public health facilities for deliveries, especially by poor households.

Distance to a facility and knowledge of the presence of community health workers (CHWs) are consistent predictors of the use of reproductive health services. A 2008 study conducted in rural Afghanistan shows that major factors affecting the use of modern contraception are exposure to media, knowledge of the presence of a CHW, household wealth, travel time to a health facility, and parity (Steinhardt and others 2009). Awareness of a CHW, household wealth, the presence of other married women in the household, travel time to a health facility, education, and perceptions of the nearest health facility significantly affect the use of skilled antenatal care. Variables that affect skilled birth attendance and institutional deliveries include all the variables that affect antenatal care except awareness of a CHW.

Health care–seeking and distance. Wealth also indirectly affects health care utilization through distance to health facilities. It is much more difficult for the poor to get to a health facility; distance is a significant obstacle to seeking care. There is evidence that health facilities tend to be located closer to better-off households and farther from poor households. Comparing travel time to the nearest health facility using households' routine mode of transportation, 13.5 percent of the poorest households live

Table 2.7   Institutional Delivery, by Wealth Quintile

		Institutional delivery		Home delivery
Wealth quintile	Delivered at an institution	Hospital	Public health clinic	Private health clinic	Own, relative's, or neighbor's home
Lowest (poorest)	3.2	2.2	1.0	0.1	96.8
Second	7.1	4.5	2.2	0.4	92.9
Middle	15.3	8.2	4.4	2.7	84.7
Fourth	19.1	13.2	3.7	2.1	80.9
Highest (richest)	33.0	24.1	5.0	3.9	67.0
Overall	14.6	9.8	3.1	1.7	85.4

Source: Afghanistan Household Survey (Ministry of Public Health 2006).

within two hours of a health facility, compared with 26.2 percent of households in the wealthiest quintile. Furthermore, 54.3 percent of households in the poorest quintile live more than six hours from a health facility, compared with only 3.8 percent of households in the wealthiest quintile. Among people who sought care for illness in the 30 days preceding the survey, 88.1 percent from the wealthiest quintile sought care when ill, compared with 65.0 percent from the poorest quintile (Steinhardt and others 2009). Distance from the facility is presumably one of the reasons behind this difference.

Immunization and distance. Children living farther from a health facility have lower immunization rates than other children (table 2.8). The immunization rate for BCG among children who live more than four hours from a health facility is only 60 percent of that of children who live less than two hours from a facility. DPT1 immunization rates for children living farthest from health facilities are 55 percent of those living closest, and the gap is even greater for DPT2 and DPT3 immunization rates.

First contact can happen when sick children are brought to a health facility. Care seeking for sick children under five may be less sensitive to travel time than the use of preventive services. For this reason, immunizations, such as BCG and DPT1, that are given at first contact are not as closely related to the distance to a health facility. Because DPT2 and DPT3 are given over multiple contacts with a health facility, children living farther away are much less likely to receive the second and third dose. The smaller gap for OPV3 and measles may be attributed to national immunization days, which reduce the distance that needs to be traveled to receive the vaccine.

Table 2.8   Effect of Distance to Health Facility on Immunization Coverage
(percentage of children 12–23 months immunized)

Distance	BCG	OPV3	DPT1	DPT2	DPT3	Measles	All vaccinations	No vaccinations
< 2 hours	78.8	74.2	68.9	56.2	41.6	69.5	33.4	10.5
≥ 2 hours but < 3 hours	59.6	63.5	50.7	42.7	28.7	48.6	20.4	19.0
≥ 3 hours but < 4 hours	65.2	69.4	54.1	39.8	24.3	63.4	17.1	13.8
≥ 4 hours	47.7	55.5	38.0	26.8	14.5	44.0	11.0	25.1
Overall	70.2	69.7	60.4	48.7	34.6	62.6	27.1	14.1

Source: Afghanistan Household Survey (Ministry of Public Health 2006).
Note: BCG = Bacillus Calmette-Guerin; DPT = diphtheria, pertussis, and tetanus; OPV = oral polio vaccine.

Reproductive health care and distance. Care seeking for reproductive health is low in Afghanistan, and utilization is a function of distance (figure 2.3). Although overall care seeking for reproductive health is low in Afghanistan, there is more than a 25 percentage point drop in the utilization of skilled birth attendance for women who live more than six hours from a health facility compared with women who live within two hours of a facility. Less than 5 percent of women giving birth who live more than six hours from a health facility have a skilled birth attendant.

The relationship between distance to a health care facility and maternal care is reflected in maternal mortality ratios, which are extremely high in remote and rural areas. Rural areas, especially remote ones, have a double problem: rural facilities are less likely to have skilled female health workers, and women who live in remote areas have more difficulty accessing health facilities.

Four representative districts were assessed in a study conducted by UNICEF and the Centers for Disease Control in 2002 (1381 AC). These districts represent a continuum of settings—from urban to remote rural—present in Afghanistan. Within each selected province, districts

Figure 2.3   Effect of Distance to Health Facility on Utilization of Skilled Birth Attendant and Antenatal Care

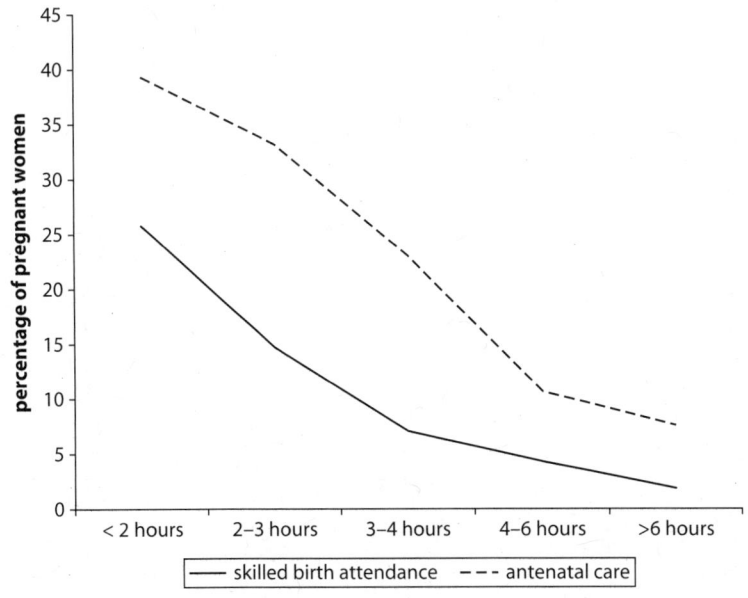

Source: Afghanistan Household Survey (Ministry of Public Health 2006).

representative of the province were chosen. In Ragh, a remote district in Badakhshan, there was 1 maternal death for every 15 childbirths. With a total fertility rate of six, the average woman in this part of Afghanistan runs more than a one in three chance of dying of maternal causes during her reproductive life (figure 2.4). This is more than 14 times the maternal mortality ratio in Kabul (418 per 100,000 live births).

Quality of Health Service Delivery

The results of annual health facility assessments show continued improvements in the quality of health service delivery across the country. The quality of service delivery is measured using the Balanced Score Card, an index generated from health facility assessments that measure 26 key components of the delivery of basic health services.

The annual national health facility assessment has been evaluating the quality of health service delivery since 2004 (1383 AC) using the Balanced Score Card. The survey covers more than 600 facilities each year, with about 6,000 patient-provider interactions and exit interviews and about 2,000 health care provider interviews. The scorecard includes six domains: patients and community, staff, capacity for service provision, service provision, financial systems, and overall MOPH vision (the components of each of these domains are summarized in appendix A).

The mean score of the Balanced Score Card improved steadily between 2004 (1383 AC) and 2008 (1387 AC), rising from 50.4 to 71.1 (table 2.9).

Figure 2.4   Maternal Mortality Ratio in Four Districts in Afghanistan, 1999–2002 (1378–81 AC)

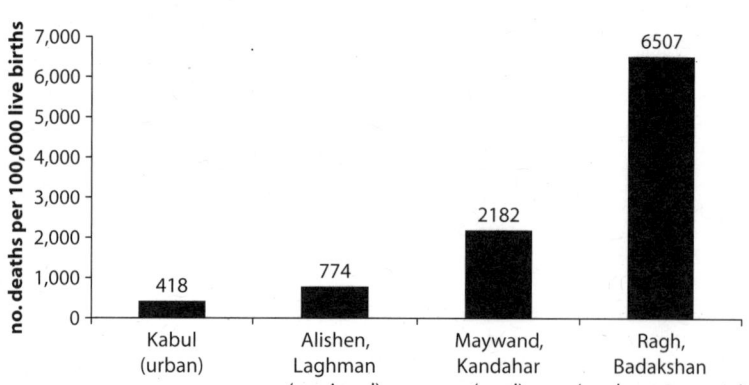

Source: Bartlett and others 2005.

**Table 2.9   Mean Balanced Score Card
Score, 2004–08 (1383–87 AC)**

Year	Score
2004	50.4
2005	57.1
2006	61.8
2007	69.0
2008	71.7

Source: Afghanistan Health Sector Balanced Score Card
(Ministry of Public Health 2008a).

Some of the factors driving these advances include the increased availability of essential drugs and family planning supplies, the increase in overall patient satisfaction, increased delivery care for pregnant women, improved equipment and laboratory functionality, and increased use of health facilities for outpatient care.

CHAPTER 3

Financing of the Health Sector

Afghanistan has a high level of health spending as a share of gross domestic product (GDP), but per capita spending is low (table 3.1). Furthermore, the share of public spending in the total is less than 30 percent, and the vast majority of that is from external sources. Estimates show that the share of private spending is in the range of 76–83 percent of total spending, most of which is out of pocket (World Bank 2004; Ministry of Public Health 2006).

Increasing external assistance to health has been critical, especially for expanding the basic package of health services (BPHS). External assistance is the major source of financing the BPHS; it has enabled improvements in and expansion of publicly financed health services throughout the country. External assistance accounted for 85 percent of government expenditure during 2002/03–2007/08 (1381–86 AC). Given the fiscal constraints facing Afghanistan, external assistance is likely to remain a major source of public expenditure on health in the near future.

Lack of accurate information on the overall resource flow and spending patterns is constraining the planning process. Accurate information is lacking concerning the amount of development assistance to the health sector, private spending on health, how money is spent, and which criteria are applied in making allocation decisions. This lack of accurate data

Table 3.1   Breakdown of Health Expenditures in Selected Economies, 2007 (1386 AC)
(weighted based on 2006 population)

Economy	Per capita GDP (dollars)	Per capita health spending (dollars)	Total health spending (percentage of GDP)	Public spending (percentage of total spending)	Social security (percentage of total spending)	Private spending (percentage of total spending)	External spending (percentage of total spending)
Afghanistan	290	34.65	11.8	27.7	0	72.3	23
South Asia	475.17	140.39	5.45	23.66	8.04	76.34	2.48
Sub-Saharan Africa	487.14	119.71	5.32	39.58	1.92	60.42	17.58
Low income	423.63	115.18	5.30	29.14	6.18	70.86	7.89

Source: Ministère des Affaires Etrangères 2007.
Note: Figures for Afghanistan are median "direct" expenditures.

on spending magnitudes and patterns seriously constrains the efficient use of resources and viable health policy making.

This chapter documents the levels and sources of financial flows into the health sector in Afghanistan. It provides a comprehensive view of financial resource flows and allocations within the sector. Specifically, it provides data on the resource envelope for the sector from all sources, describes how health resources are allocated geographically and to programs and activities, examines priority setting for health expenditure, and gives an overview of the budget structure and process.

Revenue-Generation Capacity

Domestic general revenue in Afghanistan is so low that there is little room for increasing public health expenditure from domestic sources (figure 3.1). A major challenge for the government is increasing domestic revenues, which have historically been very low, growing from 4.7 percent of GDP in 2003/04 (1382 AC) to only 7.5 percent in 2006/07 (1385 AC) and then declining to 7.0 percent in 2007/08 (1386 AC). This low capacity for raising revenue is a major constraint to increasing investments in health.

As a result, Afghanistan remains heavily dependent on external assistance, limiting the government's ability to set its own priorities. Because some assistance is earmarked, some spending priorities are effectively predetermined. Within these limits, however, the government's priorities are moving away from security and toward the social sectors, including health (figures 3.2 and 3.3). The share of public spending devoted to health increased from 3 percent to 4 percent between 2007/08 (1386 AC) and 2008/09 (1387 AC).

Figure 3.1   Sources of National Budget Funds, 2007/08 (1386 AC)

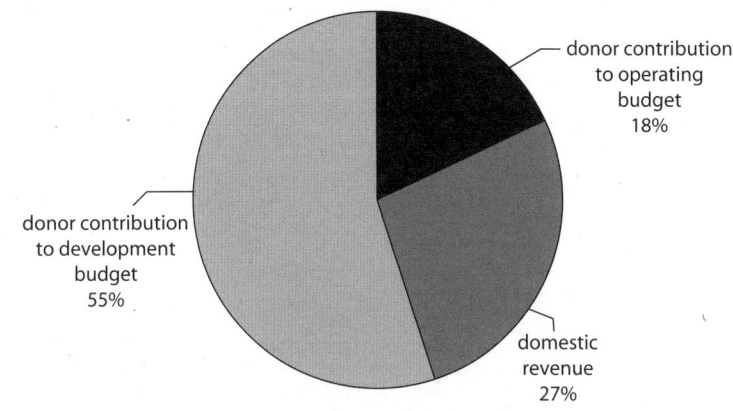

donor contribution
to operating
budget
18%

donor contribution
to development
budget
55%

domestic
revenue
27%

Source: Author's compilation.

Level and Sources of Financing for the Health Sector

Funding for the health sector comes from three sources: the government, external donors, and out-of-pocket payments by patients. This section looks at the levels of and trends in all three sources of funding.

Total Health Sector Financing

Total public spending on health increased from $193.1 million in 2004/05 (1383 AC) to $277.7 million in 2008/09 (1387 AC) (table 3.2). This includes both the government's core budget and external assistance, which represents more than 85 percent of total public spending on health.[1]

Per capita public spending on health increased from $8.06 in 2005/06 (1384 AC) to $10.92 in 2008/09 (1387 AC) (table 3.3). With annual population growth of 2 percent, Afghanistan saw nominal per capita public expenditure on health increase by 36.5 percent over this period.

When actual health service coverage is taken into account, annual per capita spending was as high as $18.20 in 2008/09 (1387 AC). The coverage of health services was examined to better understand how much is actually spent per capita on service delivery. Two elements were considered: the coverage of BPHS contracts, estimated at 80 percent for 2008/09 (1387 AC),[2] and the population living within two hours' walking distance from a facility, estimated at about 60 percent. As coverage increases without proportional increases in finance, effective per capita spending is bound to fall.

Figure 3.2   Total Public Spending (Core and External) by Sector, 2007/08 (1386 AC) and 2008/09 (1387 AC)

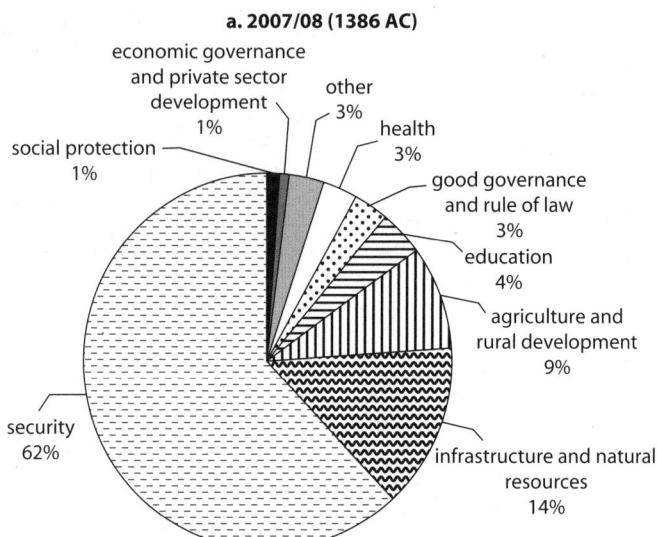

a. 2007/08 (1386 AC)

economic governance
and private sector
development
1%

other
3%

social protection
1%

health
3%

good governance
and rule of law
3%

education
4%

agriculture and
rural development
9%

security
62%

infrastructure and natural
resources
14%

b. 2008/09 (1387 AC)

economic governance and
private sector development
3%

others
3%

social protection
2%

health
4%

good governance
and rule of law
5%

education
9%

security
41%

agriculture and
rural development
10%

infrastructure and natural
resources
23%

Source: Author's compilation.

Figure 3.3   External Budget by Sector, 2008/09 (1387 AC)

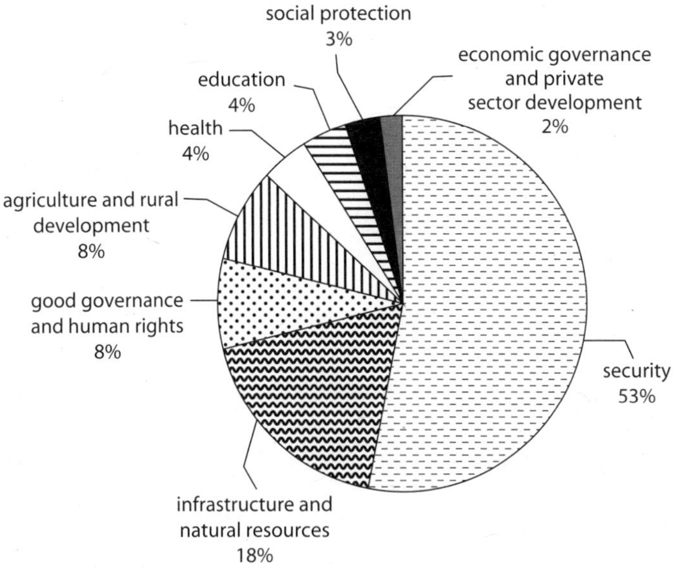

Source: Author's compilation.

Table 3.2   Total Public Funding on the Health Sector, 2004/05–2008/09 (1383–87 AC)
(millions of dollars)

Category	2004/05 (1383 AC)	2005/06 (1384 AC)	2006/07 (1385 AC)	2007/08 (1386 AC)	2008/09 (1387 AC)
External assistance	138.4	165.5	198.8	220.7	223.5
Operating budget	25.2	27.4	27.6	30.7	27.7
Total funding	163.6	192.9	226.4	251.4	251.2
With discretionary funding (development budget)	163.6[a]	193.1	231.1	258.4	277.7

Source: Author's compilation.
a. Data on the level of discretionary budget were not available for this year.

Table 3.3   Total and per Capita Public Expenditure on Health, 2005/06–2008/09 (1384–87 AC)
(millions of dollars, except where stated otherwise)

Item	2005/06 (1384 AC)	2006/07 (1385 AC)	2007/08 (1386 AC)	2008/09 (1387 AC)
Total funding	193.1	231.1	258.4	277.7
Population	24.0	24.4	24.9	25.4
Funding per capita	8.1	9.5	10.4	10.9
With 80% coverage	10.17	11.8	13.0	13.7
With 60% coverage	13.4	15.8	17.3	18.2

Source: Author's compilation.

External Assistance

External assistance to the sector has increased steadily, reaching its peak of $223.5 million in 2008/09 (1387 AC)(see table 3.2). External assistance, which is the main source of finance to the sector, has increased by a factor of 2.4 since 2003/04 (1382 AC). After an initial sharp increase in the immediate postconflict period, increases in external assistance have leveled off (figure 3.4).[3] This leveling off is attributed mainly to a decrease in the construction budget supported by the U.S. Agency for International Development (USAID).

Contribution by donor. The largest donors to the health sector are the United States, the European Community, the United Nations, and the World Bank (figure 3.5). Excluding the United Nations, these donors now support more than 90 percent of primary health care expenditures. The largest share of UN assistance is allocated to immunization programs, which represent 47 percent of UN assistance. The data do not include Provincial Reconstruction Team construction activities other than those funded by the United States.

A number of bilateral actors disengaged from the health sector in 2003/04 (1382 AC) because of financial constraints and because the emergency phase was presumed finished.[4] As a result, although "other bilateral donors" and the United Nations provided a larger portion of the contribution in the immediate postconflict era, the relative contributions

Figure 3.4   Trends in External Assistance to the Health Sector, 2003/04–2008/09 (1382–87 AC)

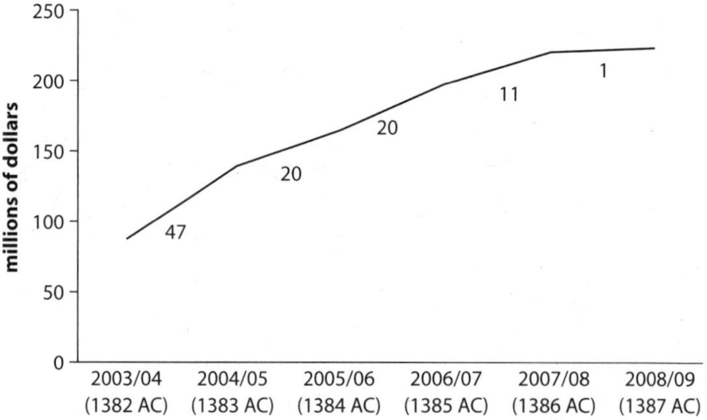

Source: Author's compilation.

Figure 3.5   Donor Contributions to External and Nondiscretionary Development Budget, 2004/05–2008/09 (1383–87 AC)

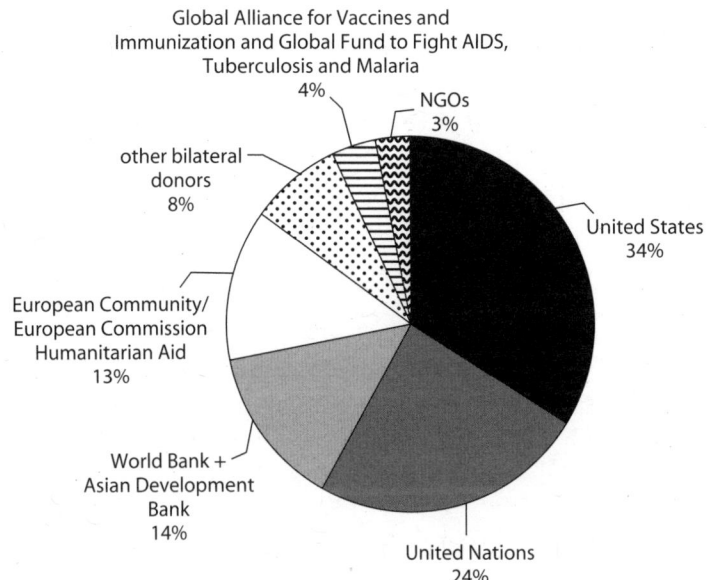

Global Alliance for Vaccines and Immunization and Global Fund to Fight AIDS, Tuberculosis and Malaria 4%

NGOs 3%

other bilateral donors 8%

United States 34%

European Community/ European Commission Humanitarian Aid 13%

World Bank + Asian Development Bank 14%

United Nations 24%

Source: Author's compilation.

of donors to the health sector did not substantially vary between 2004/05 and 2008/09 (1387 AC). The "nongovernmental organization" (NGO) contribution is, in fact, mostly bilateral funding channeled through NGOs, plus some self-financed NGOs, such as the Aga Khan Foundation and the International Committee of the Red Cross.

The proportion of funding received from the Global Alliance for Vaccines and Immunization (GAVI) and the Global Fund to Fight AIDS, Tuberculosis and Malaria (GFATM) is much lower than in most developing countries, for two reasons. First, the magnitude of other external assistance dwarfs the contribution of these two sources. Second, Afghanistan just started tapping these sources of funding. The proportion is likely to increase in the coming years, as a result of implementation of new GFATM grants and the Health Systems Strengthening grant from GAVI, which started only in 2008/09 (1387 AC).

Trends in donor contributions. It appears that assistance from all donors may have reached its peak (figure 3.6). For some donors, levels of assistance rose during the initial years, reached a peak, and then started a

Figure 3.6   Trends in Assistance by Main External Contributors to the Health Sector, 2003/04–2008/09 (1382–87 AC)

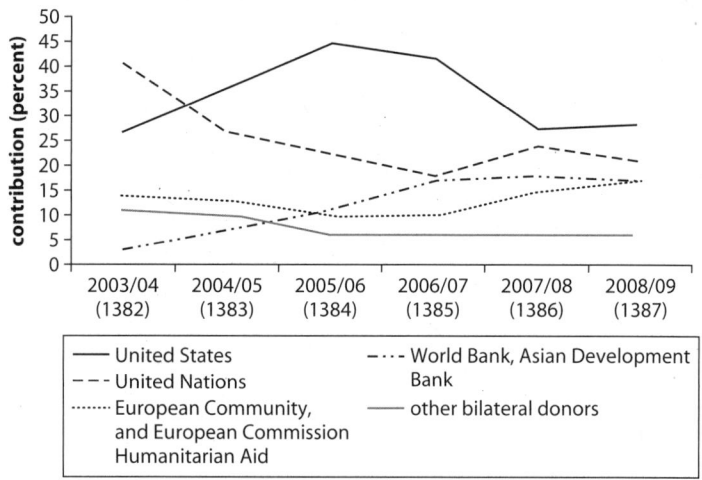

Source: Author's compilation.

downward movement. For other donors, support levels rose consistently and then remained steady at their peak level. The level of support among all donors stopped rising in 2007/08 (1386 AC).

Out-of-Pocket Payments

Afghanistan has no health insurance or prepayment system; private expenditure on health is thus entirely from out-of-pocket payments made at the time of service use. The following discussion uses data from the Afghanistan Household Survey (Ministry of Public Health 2006) to estimate this expenditure.

The survey, conducted in 2006 (1385 AC), finds that 79.9 percent of individuals who reported illness sought care outside the home and 99 percent of them paid for health care. The median spent was $10 per illness episode. Based on that expenditure, the median per capita out-of-pocket health expenditure is $14 a year. Annual per capita mean private expenditure was $36, after excluding the six outliers in the study with expenditures of $2,000 and above. (When all cases are included, annual mean per capita expenditure rises to $69 a year.) After deducting food, lodging, and transportation costs, the annual median per capita "direct" private health expenditure was $9.80 and the mean was $25.50. As in most other low-income countries, drugs and supplies dominate out-of-pocket health expenditures (40 percent), with transportation costs accounting for the next largest share (19 percent) (figure 3.7). Consultation fees make up only 14 percent of total out-of-pocket expenditures.

Estimated annual public spending on health was $9.45 per capita in 2006/07 (1385 AC). This figure includes both the government's own funding sources and external sources spent directly by and channeled through the government. Total per capita health expenditure was therefore $23.45–$45.45. If only direct health expenditures are included (without expenditures for food and transportation), per capita health expenditure was $19.25–$34.65.[5] This is a large amount compared with the annual per capita cost of the World Health Organization's "minimum package of essential health services" ($15–$30) for low-income countries. In fact, the estimate would likely have been higher than indicated here if the Afghanistan Household Survey had covered urban areas. By excluding urban areas, where the private sector is prominent, the survey underestimates expenditures made by users of private sector health services. If urban residents are, on average, better off than rural residents, the survey further underestimates overall out-of-pocket expenditures.

Private out-of-pocket expenditure represents 72–79 percent of total expenditures on health (table 3.4). (The mean private expenditure is

Figure 3.7   Out-of-Pocket Health Care–Related Expenditures, 2006 (1385 AC)

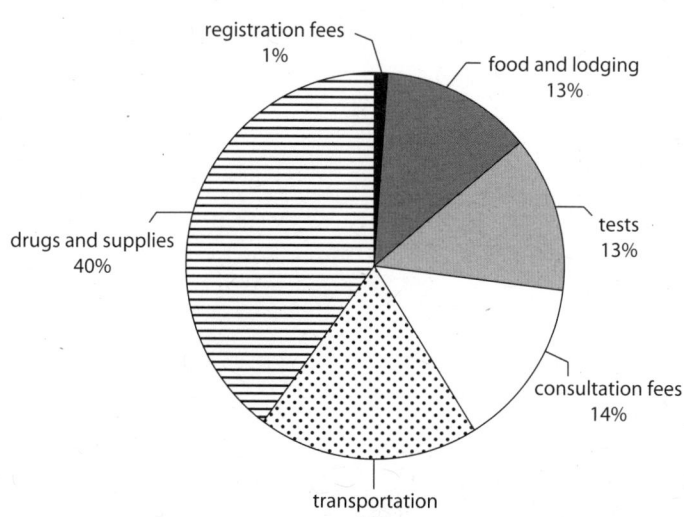

Source: Afghanistan Household Survey (Ministry of Public Health 2006).

Table 3.4   Estimated per Capita Spending on Health, 2006/07 (1385 AC)
(dollars, except where otherwise indicated)

Category	Median	Mean without outliers	Mean with outliers
Private expenditure per capita	14.0	36.0	69.0
Private direct health expenditure per capita	9.8	25.2	48.3
Public expenditure per capita	9.5	9.5	9.5
Total public + private expenditure per capita	23.5	45.5	78.5
Private/total expenditure (percent)	60.0	79.0	88.0
Total public + private direct expenditure per capita	19.3	34.7	58.0
Direct private/total expenditure (percent)	50.9	72.3	83.3

Source: Author's compilation.

72 percent if only direct medical costs are included and 79 percent of total health expenditure if all costs related to illness episodes are included.)

In the absence of health insurance, a health shock can place an enormous financial burden on households. The median expenditure for those seeking care shows that patients in the poorest income quintile have higher expenditures than patients in the wealthiest quintile ($10.00 versus $8.40).[6] This is partly because the poor may postpone seeking care and therefore have more severe illnesses that are more costly to treat. Moreover, the poor are likely to live farther away from health facilities and incur higher transportation costs. The burden is much higher when people who fail to seek care—either because it is too expensive (23.5 percent) or because places for treatment are too far away (26.5 percent)—are also taken into account.

User fees constitute a small share of out-of-pocket expenditures (see figure 3.7). The largest share of out-of-pocket payments is the cost of drugs and supplies. Consultation and registration fees make up only 15 percent of the total. When user fees include only consultation and registration fees, abolishing user fees may not have the intended impact of reducing out-of-pocket expense.

Concerned with financial barriers to access to health care services, the government abolished user fees for BPHS facilities in 2008 (1387 AC). However, there is no systematic evidence in the literature that abolishing user fees at public health facilities substantially reduces households' out-of-pocket expenditures. This may be because of a combination of the small share of user fees in total out-of-pocket payments and the possible increase in utilization following the removal of user fees. Reports of the increase in utilization reported by NGOs after fees were abolished need to be carefully documented with reliable supporting data.

Moreover, although formal fees have been abolished, informal payments continue to be made at public facilities that are supposed to be free. This practice is common in Afghanistan, as in many countries, especially in hospitals. One preliminary report on the Central Hospital in Kabul reported an escalation of corruption within the hospital, as evidenced by the number of staff being paid for services by patients. Estimates show that 80 percent of patients pay hospital staff informally (Loma Linda University 2008).

Expenditure Priorities

This section examines expenditures priorities in the sector. It describes funding by program, activity, and geographic area.

Financing by Program

Allocation of health resources by program has been relatively constant over the years, reflecting the government's priorities (figure 3.8). Within the health budget, a large share is allocated to primary health care and hospital service delivery through the BPHS and the essential package of hospital services (EPHS) and to communicable diseases. This is in line with what is known about the burden of disease in Afghanistan. The establishment of the BPHS and EPHS, together with the commitment of all the major stakeholders in the system, has been instrumental in maintaining a steady flow of funding for the delivery of these priority health services.

With the introduction of program budgeting in 2008/09 (1387 AC), the budget share of the hospital sector increased and now stands on a par with that for primary health care (30 percent) (figure 3.9). This increase in the hospital budget to the level of that of primary health care should be evaluated in light of the stated intention of the health sector strategy.

Expenditures on immunization dominate spending on communicable diseases, representing 60 percent of this category. Given the massive investments that this sector has attracted, the performance of these immunization programs may need a thorough assessment. Measles immunization coverage stood at about 60 percent in 2004/05 (1383 AC). Although it increased slightly in 2005/06 (1384 AC), it is still below the threshold required to prevent epidemics. This coverage has been achieved through emergency immunization campaigns, which absorbed the majority of funding before 2006/07

Figure 3.8   Trends in Allocation of Health Care Budget by Program, 2003/04–2008/09 (1382–87 AC)

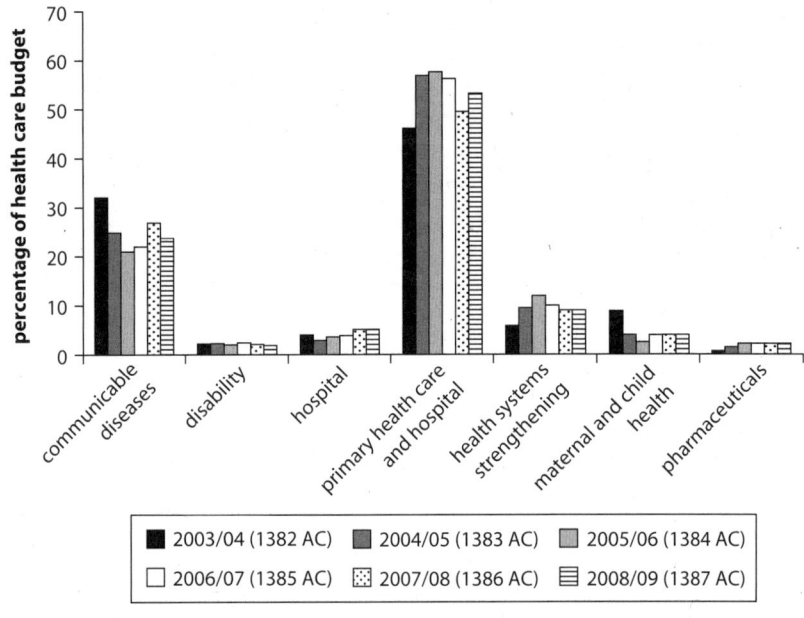

Source: Author's compilation.

Figure 3.9   Allocation of Health Care Budget by Program, 2008/09 (1387 AC)

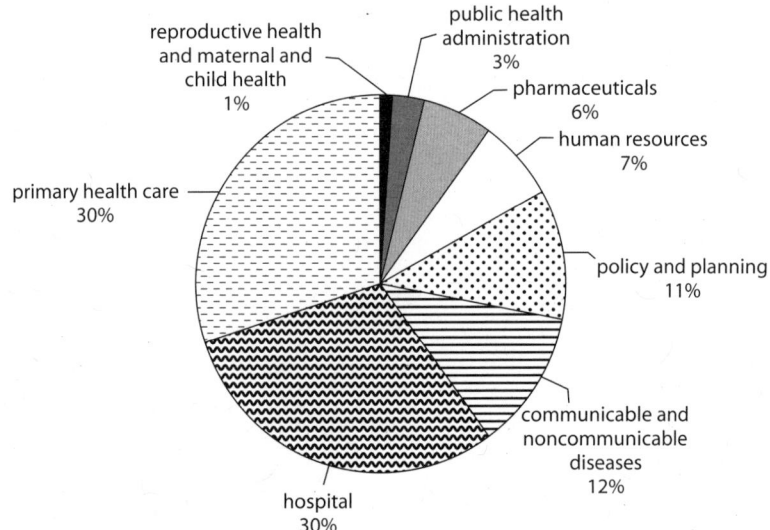

Source: Author's compilation.

(1385 AC). Routine activities, as distinct from campaigns, represented 60 percent of the immunization budget in 2007/08 (1386 AC) and 2008/09 (1387 AC). Although concrete data are not available, most stakeholders acknowledge that such campaigns are major cost drivers.

More-focused spending is needed to further expand basic health services in rural Afghanistan. Although service coverage has expanded in the past few years, the percentage of the population that is benefiting remains low. A reported 60 percent of the rural population lives more than an hour's travel time from any facility, and the coverage of key health promotion and services is low by international standards. In particular, although the number of health facilities with at least one female health worker has risen, coverage varies widely across provinces and remains largely below the level required to ensure that essential services for women are delivered.

Preliminary estimates show that about 20 percent of external funding has been allocated to the hospital sector; as the Ministry of Public Health (MOPH) starts to focus on hospitals, this figure is likely to increase[7] (figure 3.10). Notably, the construction of hospitals in various parts of the country with bilateral assistance will increase the demand for additional resources for the hospital sector, which may therefore absorb a disproportionate share of resources in the future. This pattern has already started to show up in the new budget.

Figure 3.10   Cumulative Allocation of External and Development Assistance by Program, 2003/04–2008/09 (1382–87 AC)

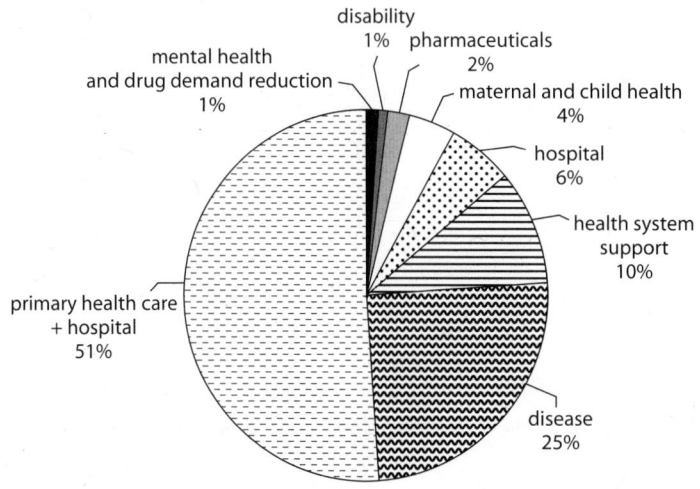

Source: Author's compilation.

No shift of aid assistance toward disease-specific vertical programs has been observed since 2003 (1382 AC). Expenditure on tuberculosis represented 8 percent of spending on communicable diseases over the 2003/04–2008/09 (1382–87 AC) period.[8] Other communicable disease programs targeted malaria, avian influenza, and leishmaniasis. Until relatively recently, spending on HIV/AIDS was very low, as program implementation started only in 2007. GFATM's first grant was allocated to health sector support, and subsequent grants for tuberculosis and malaria control were not very large compared with the BPHS and EPHS programs.

Health system support has received a stable share of external resources, focused on technical assistance and capacity building.[9] Investments in capacity building are critical given the limited absorptive capacity of the health system. The share of support dedicated to health systems strengthening is significant, and a large share of support goes to technical assistance. Such expenditures are better allocated if the ministry assesses and prioritizes areas where technical assistance is needed and there is a need to build in-house capacity.

Financing by Activity

The largest share of spending goes to health service delivery (figures 3.11 and 3.12).[10] Despite some large construction and renovation programs that are included in the spending amount, the share made up of infrastructure

Figure 3.11   Distribution of External Assistance by Activity, 2003/04–2008/09 (1382–87 AC)

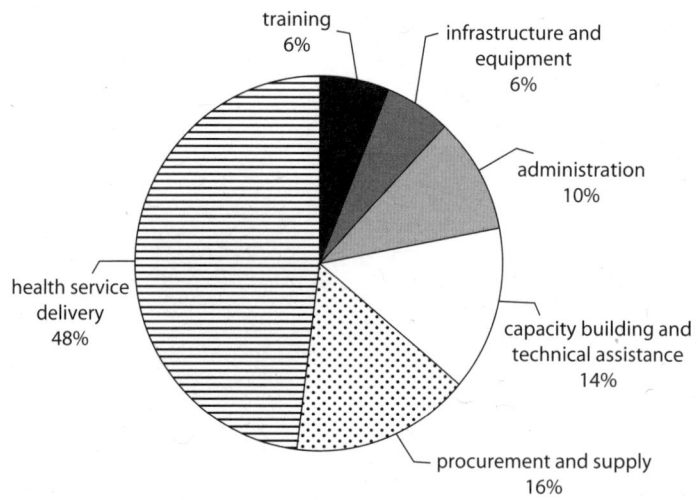

Source: Author's compilation.

Figure 3.12   Trends in Distribution of Health Care Funding by Main Activity, 2003/04–2008/09 (1382–87 AC)

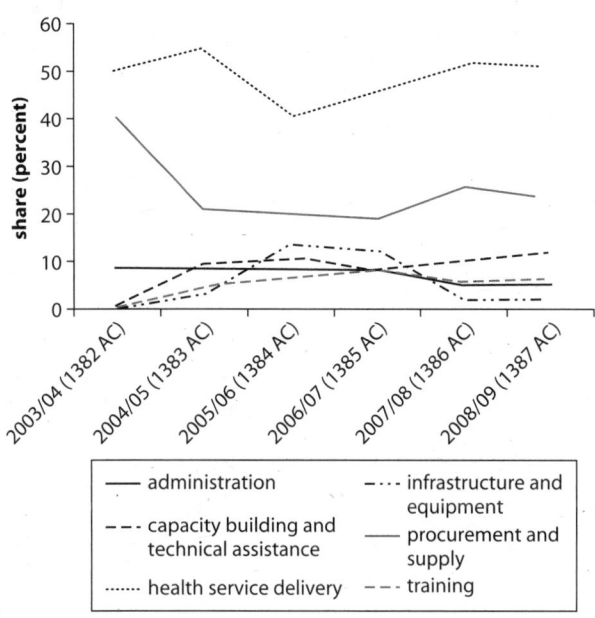

Source: Author's compilation.

and equipment spending is relatively small. The share for administration is estimated at 17–20 percent. Considering the high transactions cost environment in which the health system operates, these total costs are not particularly high. The MOPH should be credited for its focus on service delivery.

There is no clear trend in the movement of the different categories of cost between 2003/04 and 2008/09 (1382–87 AC) (see figure 3.12). However, in 2005/06–2006/07, although the share of expenditures on procurement and health delivery dipped to their minimum, those for infrastructure reached their maximum. The peak observed in infrastructure activities reflected large U.S.–funded construction and rehabilitation projects.

Within the BPHS, the largest share of spending goes to salaries and wages (39–67 percent). This share is smallest in MOPH Strengthening Mechanism provinces and largest in USAID–supported provinces.[11] The share of pharmaceuticals and medical supplies is 27–38 percent. Administrative and management costs vary greatly among donors, from 5 percent to 14 percent.

Financing by Geographic Area

Based on per capita resource allocation, no clear targeting of provinces with poor health indicators is evident (table 3.5). There are very large disparities in per capita amounts of total aid received ($8.97–$46.25). The allocation of total aid funding does not appear to be related to health need. Higher allocations for remote provinces or provinces with poor health indicators were not observed.[12]

There is no strong correlation between the aid received and the availability of health services. In the analysis, aid received per capita is compared with the relative availability of health services in rural areas, as assessed by the household survey. Provinces with the highest relative availability scores are Logar, Nangarhar, Kapisa, and Kabul; the provinces with the lowest scores are Sari Pul, Nuristan, Samangan, and Badghis. It might be expected that more resources would be allocated to the neediest provinces. Although two of the worst-performing provinces (Nuristan and Samangan) are indeed in the top quintile of aid per capita, another poor-performing province, Badghis, is in the lowest quintile of aid per capita. Similarly, a high-performing province, Logar, is among the top six provinces receiving the most aid per capita. Better targeting of future allocations should take into account the current variations in the availability of services in the provinces.

No correlation was observed between aid per capita and the operating budget. The MOPH operating budget is not being reoriented toward provinces that receive less aid. There are large variations across provinces in the levels of per capita operating budget allocated (table 3.6). They range from $0.17 to $2.62 per capita a year and are not related to the level of aid received.

Table 3.5   Total Assistance Received per Capita, by Province 2003/04–2008/09 (1382–87 AC)

(dollars)

Spending	Province
10–19	Badghis, Herat, Helmand, Baghlan, Faryab, Daykundi, Kandahar, Balkh, Nangarhar, Wardak, Khost
19–25	Paktia, Panjshir, Takhar, Kapisa, Parwan, Ghor, Farah, Sari Pul, Badakshan, Jawzjan, Paktika, Oruzgan
25–35	Ghazni, Kunar, Kunduz, Zabul, Logar, Laghman
More than 35	Nimroz, Bamyan, Samangan, Nuristan

Source: Author's compilation.

Table 3.6   Average Operating Budget per Capita, by Province, 2004/05–2008/09 (1383–87 AC)

(dollars)

Spending	Province
0.17–0.30	Paktika, Helmand, Ghazni, Daykundi, Khost, Sari Pul, Ghor, Kabul, Wardak, Takhar, Faryab
0.30–0.50	Badghis, Paktia, Kunar, Bamyan, Zabul, Logar, Badakshan, Samangan, Laghman, Oruzgan, Farah, Herat, Kunduz, Baghlan
0.60–1.0	Nangarhar, Nuristan, Kandahar, Nimroz
1.20–1.50	Balkh, Jawzjan
More than 1.6	Kapisa, Parwan, Panjshir

Source: Author's compilation.
Note: National average = 0.58. National median = 0.36.

Table 3.7   Urban Population as a Percentage of Total Population, 2005 (1384 AC)

Percentage of population in urban areas	Province
More than 20	Kabul, Baghlan, Kunduz, Jawzjan, Herat, Kandahar, Nimroz, Balkh
15–19	Nangarhar, Takhar
10–14	Parwan, Samangan, Faryab
5–10	Sari Pul, Farah, Helmand
Less than 5	Kapisa, Wardak, Logar, Ghazni, Paktika, Paktia, Khost, Kunar, Laghman, Badakshan, Badghis, Zabul, Oruzgan, Ghor, Bamyan, Daykundi, Panjshir, Nuristan

Source: Author's compilation.

There is some evidence that more aid per capita is channeled to rural and poor areas (table 3.7). Although there is well-documented evidence of disparities in poverty and access to health between rural and urban residents, the level of aid does not reflect these differences.[13] For instance, provinces in which the population is more urbanized do not receive more aid per capita than provinces that are more rural. The proportion of urban population is highest in Kabul province (79.5 percent), yet Kabul province receives among the lowest aid per capita. The proportion of urban population is greater than 20 percent in seven provinces, including Baghlan, Kunduz, and Herat, but they receive much less aid per capita than the national average. Such is not the case for provinces such as Balkh and Jawzjan, which have higher aid per capita but the same proportion of urban population as the former three provinces. In contrast, Kapisa and Punisher, where less than 5 percent of the population lives in urban areas, receive the highest aid per capita in Afghanistan.

Budget Process and Structure

This section looks at the way in which the health sector budget is structured, prepared, and implemented. It then describes the composition of expenditures in the operating budget.

Budget Structure

Afghanistan's national budget has two components: a core budget and an external budget. The core budget includes all funds flowing through the government's accounts. Within the core budget, expenditures are divided into operating and development categories. Operating expenditures are primarily recurrent and include all civil servants' wages and pensions, plus goods and services for operations and maintenance. This category also includes small investment expenditures. Both government revenues and external aid, notably grants through the Afghanistan Reconstruction Trust Fund (ARTF) and the Law and Order Trust Fund for Afghanistan (LOTFA), finance these expenditures.

Development expenditures primarily include investments in capital goods (for example, building facilities); it also includes a substantial portion of recurrent expenditures, such as technical assistance, training, and on-budget grants. These expenditures are financed through direct budget support and external project assistance channeled through the budget. External project assistance consists mainly of projects funded by the World Bank and Asian Development Bank, as well as investment projects financed by the ARTF. New commitments for health care from the U.S. government are also expected to be channeled through this budget.

The external budget comprises all external assistance funds not flowing through the government accounts, including those directly disbursed by donors. External budget expenditures include technical assistance, most capital expenditures, and significant donor-financed recurrent expenditures. Support for the BPHS and EPHS from the European Commission and USAID, as well as most bilateral assistance, is also included in this budget.

The health budget is managed by two departments with separate lines of reporting and weak coordination. Within the MOPH, two units from different general directorates report to different deputy ministers to manage the budget. The Health Care Financing Department of the Policy and Planning General Directorate (GDPP) oversees the development budget, and the Finance and Accounting Directorate of the Administration General

Directorate oversees the operating budget. The two departments do not seem to coordinate their work adequately.

The introduction of a program budgeting exercise provides an opportunity to unify the preparation of the operating and development budgets. Program budgeting was introduced by the Ministry of Finance in 2007/08 to link the national sectoral strategy with the annual budget and prioritize allocations. The 2008/09 (1387 AC) health budget comprises eight major programs, which are linked mainly to the departmental structures of the MOPH. Program budgeting is an important step toward better alignment of the priorities stated in the Afghanistan national development strategy.

Budget Preparation

The MOPH budget preparation process is complex. The MOPH receives its budget envelope for the following year from the Ministry of Finance at the end of July. Program managers are required to evaluate their needs and prepare a detailed action plan. Output and outcome indicators, with their costs, are then discussed with program managers. Consolidation of the budget is carried out at the ministry level, with priority given to projects already being implemented with identified funding. Allocations to new projects are negotiated with the Ministry of Economy and the Ministry of Finance. A proposed budget is then presented to the Ministry of Finance in October.

The current preparation process is characterized by the following:

- *Tight schedule for budget preparation.* The current schedule, with budget ceilings communicated late in the process, allows little time for units to prepare their budgets, seriously limiting the opportunity for substantive analysis and discussion. The process results in poor prioritization, a result of lack of time for consultations. Ceilings for the development budget depend on the donor financial review, carried out twice a year by the Aid Coordination Unit of the Budget Department in the Ministry of Finance.

- *Lack of consultation in the development of the operating budget.* The General Directorate of Administration prepares the operating budget; very little consultation is involved in this process. Program managers have little information about their budgets and are not involved in their preparation. The budget is developed for the entire ministry without a breakdown by programs. At the provincial level, it is not possible to

separate the provincial health office budget from the hospital budget
in provinces in which the hospital is under neither the EPHS nor the
Hospital Reform Program.

• *Weak data for costing.* The basis for costing activities is weak, as programs have little information on their budgets, the expenditure tracking
system is not fully implemented in the MOPH, and the data on the
health sector do not allow a bottom-up costing. This is a major issue,
notably for program budgeting.

Budget Implementation

Execution rates of the development budget are very low (table 3.8). This
problem is not specific to the health sector; low execution rates are perva-
sive throughout the government. At 62 percent in 2007/08 (1386 AC),
the execution rate for discretionary funds (that is, funds not earmarked
for specific projects) in the development budget was higher than the
execution rate of nondiscretionary funds, which stood at 42 percent.
There is no clear pattern for implementation rates, although health care
delivery programs tend to achieve good execution rates in general. Among
projects with less than 40 percent implementation in 2007/08 (1386 AC),
21 percent were under "health system support" (mostly technical assistance
to the MOPH) and 37 percent were under "hospital."

Weak budget execution is partly responsible for the fluctuations in the
budget. Slow budget execution may have accounted for most of the
sharp increase in the development budget between 2006/07 (1385 AC)
and 2007/08 (1386 AC) (table 3.9). When budgets are unspent, they
tend to be carried over to the next budget period and may show up, mis-
leadingly, as increases in the actual budget. The budget is reviewed by
midyear, and corrections are made to allocations. When ministries fail to

Table 3.8   Execution Rate of Core Budget, 2005/06–2007/08 (1384–86 AC)
(percent)

Budget item	2005/06 (1384 AC)	2006/07 (1385 AC)	2007/08 (1386 AC)
Operating budget for health	92	96	99
Development budget for health	65	52	51[a]
Development budget for whole government	44	54	60

Source: Treasury Department 2007/08 (1386 AC).
a. As of August 2008. The final rate is expected to be about 58 percent.

Table 3.9   Operating and Development Budget of the MOPH, 2004/05–2008/09 (1383–87 AC)

(millions of dollars)

Year	Core operating budget	Core development budget
2004/05 (1383 AC)	25.2	22.3
2005/06 (1384 AC)	27.4	31.3
2006/07 (1385 AC)	27.64	77.91
2007/08 (1386 AC)	30.7	103.5
2008/09 (1387 AC)	27.7	61.6

Source: Author's compilation.

demonstrate the capacity to absorb their funding, the cabinet considers reallocating their funds.

The midyear review has improved the quality of budget management across the government. It has allowed transparent adjustments during the year and created a feedback loop from one year's budget implementation to the next year's budget preparation.

The main reasons behind low budget execution are inefficient procurement procedures and flow of funds:

- Procurement is highly centralized and slow. At the central level, two units under two general directorates in the MOPH conduct procurement: the Health Economics and Finance Department (HEFD) of the Policy & Planning General Directorate and the Directorate for Provision and Procurement (DPP) of the Administration General Directorate. HEFD focuses on procuring services funded under the development budget; DPP procures goods and supplies support under the operating budget. The procedures are extremely slow and bureaucratic, requiring numerous authorizations and signatures (for details, see chapter 7).

- The flow of funds is also inefficient. Departments and hospitals do not have separate budgets and are not fully informed of their budgets. Work also remains to be done to ensure that service delivery units in the MOPH receive the resources and information necessary to perform their operations. One of the major issues identified is the absence of individual operating budget for programs, notably provincial hospitals. Central hospitals have no information on their budgets, which come entirely from the operating budget. Furthermore, allotments may change during the year, and hospitals are rarely informed about their allotments.

Figure 3.13   Wages and Salaries as a Share of the Operating Budget of the Ministry of Public Health and the Government of Afghanistan, 2005/06–2007/08 (1384–86 AC)

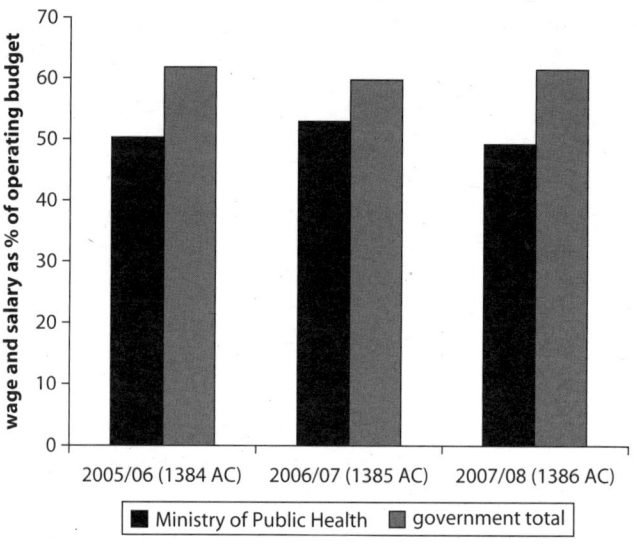

Source: Author's compilation.

Figure 3.14   Composition of the Operating Budget of the Ministry of Public Health, 2005/06–2008/09 (1384–87 AC)

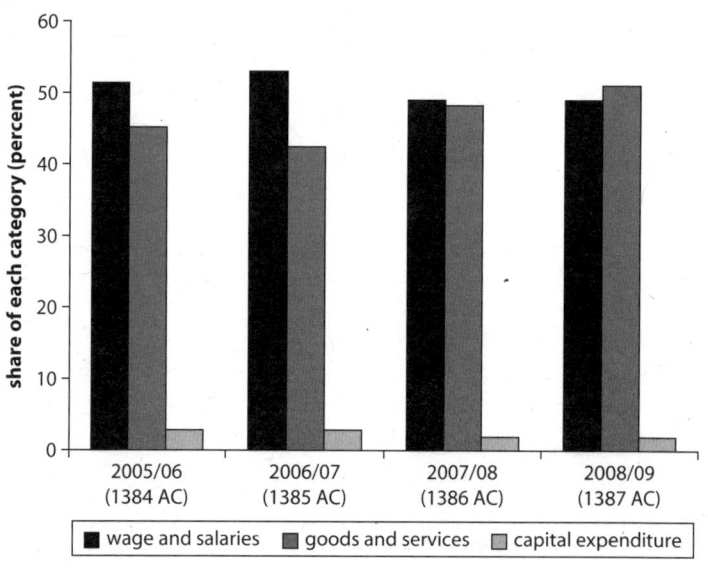

Source: Author's compilation.

Structure of Expenditures in the Operating Budget

Unlike in other ministries or other national budgets, wages and salaries in Afghanistan's Ministry of Health do not constrain the operating budget. Although a key driver of spending in the national operating budget in general is wages and salaries, the budgets for these items do not appear to be driving the budget in the health sector, where wages and salaries in the health sector account for less than 50 percent of the operating budget (figure 3.13).[14] The fact that primary health care services are delivered by contracted agents may be part of the reason, although contracting does not explain the increase in the share of goods and services between 2005/06 and 2008/09 (1384–87 AC) (figure 3.14).

Concluding Remarks: Findings and Recommendations

Key Findings

Public spending on health increased 54 percent between 2004/05 and 2008/09 (1383–87 AC), from $163.6 million to $277.7 million. At $10.92 per capita, however, it remains low. The level of spending compares favorably with neighboring South Asian countries but poorly with other developing countries. If the intention is to provide universal primary health care free of charge, the current level of spending falls short of recommended levels, which range from $15 to $30 per capita.

Much of the increase in public spending reflects increases in external assistance, which rose consistently over the period, increasing by 61.5 percent (from $138.4 million to $223.5 million). Meanwhile, although the government's budget allocation for health increased in absolute terms, it decreased in relative terms, falling from 5.1 percent of total government spending in 2005/06 (1384 AC) to 4.0 percent in 2008/09 (1387 AC).

The share of private expenditures ranges from 72 percent to 79 percent of total expenditure on health. Median per capita private health expenditure in 2006 (1385 AC) was $14 a year, and mean spending was $36. This level of spending represents 5–12 percent of per capita income.

Although the execution rate of the core operating budget increased from 92 percent in 2005/06 (1384 AC) to 99 percent in 2007/08 (1387 AC), the execution rate of the core development budget remains below

60 percent. Primary health care programs tend to achieve higher implementation rates in general, while technical assistance and construction projects have lagged behind. The main reasons identified for these low implementation rates are poor internal and external coordination and inefficient procurement processes.

Construction programs have suffered from particularly poor execution rates. As discussed in chapter 5, budget execution for construction programs has been poor. This may be because there are some risks linked with any increase in infrastructure capacity that creates large liabilities for future operation and maintenance.[15]

Spending patterns have been well matched to health priorities, as stated in the Afghanistan national development strategy. The majority of financial support is allocated and spent on primary health care programs and communicable diseases, particularly immunization. The BPHS and EPHS have been powerful tools for both harmonizing donor support and keeping the focus on the delivery of essential services instead of vertical programs. The BPHS, the central conduit for primary health care in Afghanistan, received a steadily increasing share of external assistance (24 percent in 2003/04 [1382 AC] and 42 percent in 2008/09 [1387 AC]). The Expanded Program on Immunization (EPI) has received a large and stable share of funding from UN agencies and bilateral donors. Other communicable diseases (especially tuberculosis, malaria, and leishmaniasis but also avian influenza) have attracted less funding, although the implementation of new GFATM grants is expected to sharpen the focus on vertical programs.

Maternal and child health is receiving additional direct funding from donors but a very small share of the government budget. To continue to reduce maternal and infant mortality, Afghanistan needs to increase its skilled female workforce in the sector. Donors are funding some training programs and institutions to increase the number of midwives, particularly community midwives. This funding is part of technical assistance and capacity building projects classified under "health system strengthening" or "primary health care." This effort will have to be sustained in order to counterbalance the social and cultural barriers and security issues that are currently preventing more female staff from being deployed in rural areas.

Per capita government health expenditure varies widely across provinces. For external assistance, it ranges from $8.97 to $46.25 a year; for operating budgets, it ranges from $0.17 to $2.62 a year. Except for supervised deliveries and skilled antenatal care, for which lower-performing provinces received higher allocations, no correlation was found between poor performance as measured by the index of health services availability, immunization coverage, and aid per capita received.

Some inequity is evident in health financing patterns, as the poorest provinces often receive less external aid per capita and the poor have large out-of-pocket expenses. In the absence of data on the distribution of health spending across population groups, equity in health care finance is assessed through three measures:

- *Per capita allocation by province.* The data show that some of the poorest provinces received less external aid per capita than some of the wealthiest ones.
- *Out-of-pocket expenditure.* The poor have large out-of-pocket expenditures.
- *Utilization of service.* One of the major barriers to access to health services is distance, and the poor are likely to live farther away from a health facility than the rich.

The poor appear to prefer private providers to public providers. According to the 2006 (1385 AC) Afghanistan Household Survey, although a higher percentage of the poor use public health facilities, a large proportion of the poor still use private providers. It is not clear why the poor prefer to use private providers to public facilities, which cost less, but it will be important to understand this pattern to address their unmet health service needs in the most affordable way.

Recommendations

Expansion of services to the more remote and poor areas of Afghanistan will depend heavily on the availability of additional financing. The availability of additional government funds for health is unlikely, so the government should analyze options for using existing resources more efficiently for expanding coverage. For example, by maintaining user fees for hospital services, with appropriate exemptions for low-income patients, it may be possible to generate additional resources to expand the BPHS to remote areas of the country.

Out-of-pocket payments. Out-of-pocket payments make up 79 percent of total spending on health; for poor families the financial burden of health shocks can be very large. Most out-of-pocket payments go toward expenditure on pharmaceuticals and supplies. The government could explore policies to reduce out-of-pocket health expenditures, such as some form of community-based insurance in partnership with private providers. (Chapter 4 shows that private providers are popular -even in rural Afghanistan.) Establishing partnerships that protect consumers from paying large out-of-pocket payments would also give the government a tool with which to monitor and regulate the sector.

Budget execution. Strengthening the absorptive capacity of the MOPH needs immediate attention. It is hard to make a case for more resources while the allocated budget is not being fully used. In this regard, improving the procurement capacity of the ministry should be made a priority.

National health account. Establishing a regular national health account system would provide a useful management tool with which to track the flow of funds through the health sector. Various donors have expressed interest in supporting the establishment of a national health account. Efforts could be coordinated with government agencies already involved in the preparation of national income accounts. The ultimate objective should be securing sufficient, predictable, and less volatile sources of finance that would allow for a meaningful policy-making exercise in line with national priorities. Obtaining accurate information on resource flows into the sector and allocation patterns, as well as comparisons with national priorities, is critical. This book provides the first systematic documentation of health sector resource sources, levels, and uses.

Notes

1. The breakdown between discretionary and nondiscretionary budget was not available for 2004/05 (1383 AC). It was therefore excluded to avoid double-counting of projects under the development budget and total aid funding. Some programs have changed budget status over the years. For example, some United Nations Children's Fund (UNICEF) assistance was included in the core development budget in 2006/07 (1385–86 AC) but reverted to the external budget, as a result of implementation issues related to the slow release of funds.

2. As of 2008/09 (1387 AC), 80 percent of the population lived in districts in which BPHS contracts are signed. Because of limitations of geographical access, financial access, and insecurity, not everyone in these districts can benefit from the availability of the BPHS; it is estimated that the BPHS reaches about 60 percent of the total population.

3. Support for the BPHS, in particular, stabilized only in 2005/06 (1384 AC).

4. The government's approach to coordinating donor support called on donors to take responsibility for specific geographic areas. These arrangements left some bilateral donors with responsibilities that their financial resources did not allow them to take on.

5. This figure was used to estimate the data in table 3.4.

6. These expenditures do not include those of people who fail to seek care.

7. This should be treated as a preliminary figure, as data on hospital expenditures are hard to identify with the current system of documentation. Because of the difficulty in separating the BPHS, the EPHS, and construction/renovation of primary health care clinics and provincial hospitals, the data presented combine primary health care and hospitals. However, when expenditures on hospitals are identified, the data are counted separately for hospitals only.

8. In 2007 (1386 AC), Afghanistan ranked 17th out of the 22 countries with the highest tuberculosis levels in the world.

9. It was not possible to disaggregate the share of resources going to the central versus the provincial level in this area.

10. The figures from the analysis of expenditures by activity should be taken as approximate rather than exact figures, because some classifications were made without clear-cut data.

11. Because of the nature of the data, only rough estimates can be discussed. Moreover, the same level of analysis was not possible for all the contracts, because the reporting requirements differ according to the financing source. In addition, as discussed earlier, the nature of costs and services included in the contracts varies by donor, with hospital services included in some contracts and pharmaceutical procurement and training costs excluded from others.

12. Only 43 percent of external assistance was clearly identified by province, of which 76 percent was spent on the BPHS and primary health care, 6 percent on the EPHS and bilateral support to hospitals, and 12 percent on construction.

13. No disaggregated urban/rural data on financing were available; the comparison was made using provincial data.

14. A typical country devotes just over 42 percent of total general government health expenditure to paying its health workforce (WHO 2006).

15. An estimated average 40 percent of the construction cost of a hospital is required to operate and maintain it properly.

CHAPTER 4

Participation of the For-Profit Private Sector in Rural Afghanistan

Health care needs in Afghanistan are immense, and the for-profit private sector has a large potential to contribute. Although only 13 of the country's 359 districts do not have basic package of health services (BPHS) facilities, potential demand for health services far exceeds supply by the public sector. The situation is especially severe for services typically provided by female health workers. The current demand for female physicians, based on BPHS staffing requirements, is more than three times the supply in the public sector. For community midwives, demand is four times the supply; for female nurses, it is almost seven times the supply (see chapter 5). These figures are testimony to the potential role of the private sector in improving access to health care services.

The government needs to work with the private sector to achieve the national objectives of expanding coverage and improving health outcomes through good-quality services. According to the 2006 (1385 AC) Afghanistan Household Survey, the private sector is providing more than 58 percent of health services (Ministry of Public Health 2006). Although the rich use the private sector more than the poor, a significant proportion of the poor also use the private sector. More than 48 percent of the poorest quintile use private sector services for their first visit. The proportion rises to 50.6 percent and 51.2 percent for the second and third visits.

Afghanistan's constitution affirms that the state encourages and protects the establishment and expansion of private medical services and health centers in accordance with the law. These laws call for a robust health care system and encourage the development of the private sector as an integral part of that system. At the sectoral level, the Health and Nutrition Sector Strategy considers private health care providers to be a vital part of the national health care system (Ministry of Public Health 2008c).

Despite the private sector's clearly recognized role, information about its structure and performance is not well documented. According to central and provincial health officials, very little information is available about the structure, size, and quality of services provided by the private sector. Obtaining such information is critical for developing effective policy to harness the sector's energy to achieve national goals. The sector currently is growing rapidly without any particular guidance or regulation. Attempts to institute regulatory and oversight activities in order to confirm the quality of pharmaceutical products or the proper training of health care workers are highly constrained by the current lack of information about the sector.

The private sector is addressed in a fragmented manner, with no single unit responsible for coordination. Four directorates of the Ministry of Public Health (MOPH) deal with the private sector: the Legislation Implementation Ensuring Department, the Pharmaceutical Affairs General Directorate, the Health Care Services Provision General Directorate, and the Afghan Public Health Institute, which are active largely in Kabul. In the provinces, pharmacy officers are in charge of inspecting pharmacies, with support from provincial health directors.

This chapter aims to fill the gap in information on the private sector, using new sets of data. The data used were generated through a small-scale survey conducted in 2008 (1387 AC) (the Afghanistan Private Providers Survey, conducted for this book) to assess the for-profit private sector in rural Afghanistan, where more than 80 percent of the nation's population lives. The survey therefore misses information on the large segment of the for-profit private sector based in urban areas. Nevertheless, the data allow users for the first time to understand the sector in rural Afghanistan. They focus on identifying types of services, the mix of private providers in rural communities, the patterns of household utilization, and the quality and service capacity (see appendix D).

The survey yields the following four key findings:

- A large portion of health services in rural Afghanistan are provided by the private sector.
- The types of services provided by the private sector are complementary to those provided by the public sector.
- Physicians in solo practice dominate the private sector.
- The quality of care among private providers needs improvement.

The remainder of this chapter is organized as follows. The next section explains the structure of the private sector. The following section discusses the demand for privately provided health care. The types of services and the quality of services provided are presented in the following section. The last two sections focus on constraints facing the sector and offer concluding remarks.

Structure of the Private Sector

The types of private providers in Afghanistan range from solo practitioners to traditional birth attendants and mullahs (table 4.1). The classification of providers is based on ownership and organizational arrangements. Seven types of private providers are identified. Of these, two types operate informally, in the sense that they do not undergo any kind of licensing process.

The majority of private providers are physicians in solo practice. This group accounts for 66 percent of total health services provided and about 90 percent of the services provided by the private sector. The second-largest private provider, physicians practicing in pharmacies, contributes only 2.2 percent of the services provided by the private sector and 2.0 percent of total health services provided.

In the public sector, no type of BPHS facility appears dominant; the three types of facilities in the public sector show much less variation. Of total health services provided, about 6 percent are provided by district hospitals, 9 percent by comprehensive health centers, and 10 percent by basic health centers.

Both the relative contribution made by the private sector and the sector's composition vary by province (see table 4.1). The contribution of the private sector varies from 61 percent in Nimroz to 87 percent of services in Badghis. In terms of composition by type, physicians in solo practice account for 96 percent of all health services in Laghman and

Table 4.1　Types of Public and Private Sector Health Providers in Five Provinces
(percentage of total services provided by providers or facilities, except where otherwise indicated)

Sector/provider	Badghis n = 547	Baghlan n = 305	Laghman n = 423	Logar[a] n = 263	Nimroz n = 333	All five provinces n = 1,871
Private sector						
Number of facilities	474	194	309	214	204	1,395
Percentage of facilities	87	64	73	81	61	75
Physicians in solo practice	76	57	96	79	51	66
Physicians who practice in pharmacies	3	4	<1	<1	0	2
Pharmacies without physician on staff	2	<1	<1	<1	2	1
Private health clinics and hospitals	<1	<1	<1	<1	5[b]	1
Nurses	<1	0	2	0	0	<1
Traditional birth attendants and midwives	1	<1	<1	<1	1	1.5
Traditional healers (including mullahs)	9	<1	<1	0	1	3
Public sector						
Number of facilities	73	111	114	49	129	476
Percentage of facilities	13	36	27	19	39	25
District hospitals	5	3	8	9	9	6
Comprehensive health centers and subcenters	7	20	9	7	2	9
Basic health centers	2	11	10	3	27	10
Health posts/community health workers	<1	1	0	0	1	<1

Source: Author, based on survey conducted for this book.

a. Figures underrepresent the number of midwives and traditional birth attendants because security threats against the survey team precluded the inclusion of female interviewers, and subsequent security problems resulted in the truncation of the survey in one of the three sample districts.

b. The tabulation of private clinics and hospitals is higher in Nimroz than elsewhere because it includes visits to Iranian providers. Apparently, Baluchis have little difficulty crossing the border for health care.

just 51 percent in Nimroz. Despite this variation, the private sector is the major service provider and is dominated by physicians in solo practice in all provinces.

Diversity in Gender, Experience, and Formal Training

On average, 24 percent of private providers have female health workers on staff. Given the importance of female workers in attracting mothers and children to health facilities, this is a significant percentage. The proportion varies significantly, however, from 8.1 percent in Laghman to 37.3 percent in Badghis (table 4.2). The gender distribution of providers does not depend on the size of the private provider sector in each province. For instance, Nimroz, where the private sector is the smallest, has one of the largest percentages of female private health service providers, while Logar, with the second-largest private sector, has one of the lowest percentages.

Private health care providers are experienced, with an average age of 43 years. Only 7 percent are under 30, and only 5 percent are over 60. There are no notable differences in age across types of providers, except that traditional birth attendants are, on average, older than all other types of providers.

More than half of private providers have relocated to villages from other locations. In addition to their age, the study captures practitioners' experience by measuring years of work experience before locating in their current village. Although there was an increase in the number of new providers, more than 57 percent had been working in their current location since 2002 (1381 AC). Physicians in solo practice and those at private health clinics or hospitals were more likely than others to have worked somewhere other than the village in which they were currently practicing; more than two-thirds (69 percent) had worked elsewhere. In contrast, only 43 percent of midwives had worked elsewhere, and only

Table 4.2   Characteristics of Private Health Care Providers in Five Provinces

Characteristic	Badghis	Baghlan	Laghman	Logar	Nimroz	All five provinces
Female (percent)	37.3	24.1	8.1	16.7	25.9	24.0
Mean age (years)	47.4	41.6	44.2	36.3	38.7	43.2
Mean time in community (years)	14.0	13.5	10.4	3.3	8.8	11.4
With formal training (percent)	30.4	96.6	97.3	92.9	81.5	71.2

Source: Author, based on survey conducted for this book.

20 percent of traditional healers and traditional birth attendants had done so. Not all mullahs involved in providing health care had worked only in the local community; about 38 percent of them had worked elsewhere.

Family reasons and demand for health services motivate providers to start private practices. An important reason for starting a practice in a village is the demand for health services; the most common reason cited, however (accounting for 57 percent), is family considerations and discussions with the *shura-i-sehie* (community health committees). Economic factors are important for about a quarter of providers; these providers were attracted by the demand for health care services. These two motivations hold for all provinces and all types of providers, with few differences evident across provinces or provider types.

More than 70 percent of private providers have formal medical training, with substantial variation by province. The level of formal training is highest (more than 90 percent) in Laghman, Baghlan, and Logar and lowest (only 30 percent) in Badghis. The figure for Badghis should be of concern, given that 87 percent of health services there are provided by the private sector.

Days and Hours Available

Four out of five private providers operate full time and are open six to seven days a week (table 4.3). About 78 percent of providers work up to eight hours, 47 percent work between five and eight hours, and 22 percent work more than eight hours a day. There are significant differences across provinces in the number of days per week and hours per day that providers are available. The proportion of private providers operating six to seven days a week is lowest in Badghis and highest in Laghman. Providers

Table 4.3   Working Days and Hours of Operation in Five Provinces
(percentage of all private providers)

Province	Days per week available		Hours per day available		
	1–5 days	6–7 days	1–4 hours	5–8 hours	> 8 hours
Badghis	41	59	44	35	11
Baghlan	14	86	26	63	11
Laghman	8	92	28	53	17
Logar	11	89	44	22	34
Nimroz	11	89	12	50	38
All five provinces	20	80	31	47	22

Source: Author, based on survey conducted for this book.

in central districts are much more likely to be open six to seven days a week than their rural counterparts (91 percent versus 64 percent). They are also more likely to follow a standard work schedule of five to eight hours a day.

In summary, physicians in solo practice dominate private providers in rural Afghanistan. Not only do they dominate the private sector, they are also the single most important provider of health services. About a quarter of private providers are female, and close to three in four have formal training in their field. More than one in five work more than eight hours a day, and four in five stay open six to seven days a week.

Demand for Services

This section describes the demand for privately provided health services and presents the distribution of the demand by income and geographic group. It also tries to gauge the magnitude of demand for services from different types of private providers and the choice between private and public providers. Where possible, it also describes payments for these services.

It appears that the private and public sectors in rural Afghanistan are complementary. The public sector is more focused on preventive care and maternal and child health; the private sector is more focused on curative care for adults.

Private providers are used primarily to meet the health care needs of adults (table 4.4). In general, it appears that households are more likely to seek public provider care for children's routine checkups (81.5 percent) than for adults' routine checkups (31.9 percent). They are also more likely to seek public provider care for children's illnesses (41.4 percent) and injuries (42.4 percent) than for adults' illnesses (28.6 percent) or injuries (35.2 percent). Hence, for child-related health services, public providers appear to be the preferred sources of services. In contrast, private providers appear to be the preferred sources of services for adult health care. There is no systematic difference between rural and central districts.

Provider Choice and Length of Stay

Newcomers to villages are less likely than long-time residents to use private providers. The average number of visits per capita to any health facility over the previous five months is 1.2. In contrast, people who have resided in the village for less than five years have a per capita visit rate of 1.0. For people who have resided in the village for more than five years,

Table 4.4   Utilization of Public and Private Providers
(percentage of all households seeking health care)

Utilization	Overall	Central districts	Rural districts
Households with sick adult (n = 594)			
Public provider	28.6 (170)	31.6 (50)	27.5 (120)
Private provider	71.4 (424)	68.4 (108)	72.5 (316)
Households with sick child (n = 510)			
Public provider	41.4 (211)	47.3 (56)	43.1 (155)
Private provider	58.6 (299)	62.7 (94)	56.9 (205)
Households seeking routine adult health care (n = 238)			
Public provider	31.9 (76)	25.8 (16)	34.1 (60)
Private provider	68.1 (162)	74.2 (46)	65.9 (116)
Households seeking routine child health care (n = 378)			
Public provider	81.5 (308)	81.5 (88)	81.5 (220)
Private provider	18.5 (70)	18.5 (20)	18.5 (50)
Households seeking adult consultation (n = 165)			
Public provider	34.5 (57)	33.9 (20)	34.9 (37)
Private provider	65.5 (108)	66.1 (39)	61.1 (69)
Households seeking adult prescription (n = 317)			
Public provider	18.6 (59)	27.1 (26)	14.9 (33)
Private provider	81.4 (258)	72.9 (70)	85.1 (188)
Households seeking antenatal/pregnancy care (n = 248)			
Public provider	46.0 (114)	46.2 (30)	45.9 (84)
Private provider	54.0 (134)	53.8 (35)	54.1 (99)
Households with injured adult (n = 125)			
Public provider	35.2 (44)	47.1 (16)	30.8 (28)
Private provider	64.8 (81)	52.9 (18)	69.2 (63)
Households with injured child (n = 92)			
Public provider	42.4 (39)	44.1 (15)	41.4 (24)
Private provider	57.6 (53)	55.9 (19)	58.6 (34)

Source: Author, based on survey conducted for this book.
Note: Number of households is shown in parentheses.

the average per capita visit rate to any facility stands at 1.3. This difference is fully accounted for by the difference in visits to private providers (0.7 for people with less than five years' residency in the village and 1.0 for those with more than five years' residency). Although such a comparison does not control for the need for treatment or the propensity of illness among newcomers and long-time residents, the difference in choice of provider is notable.

Provider Choice and Location of Providers

Visits to private providers are more likely to require travel outside the village than visits to public providers. As all of the villages surveyed were small, it is not surprising that 72 percent of the visits to health care providers required travel outside the village. Although 74 percent of visits to private providers required travel outside the village, this was true of just 64 percent of visits to public facilities. In some provinces, more than 86 percent of visits required such travel. There were significant variations among provinces. In Badghis 86.1 percent of visits to private providers and 92.3 percent of visits to public providers required travel outside the village; in Logar travel was necessary for only 29.7 percent of visits to private providers and 54.1 percent of visits to public providers.

Health Needs and Provider Choice
Private providers are the more likely choice for follow-up visits. More than three out of four visits to providers were for a new illness (76 percent), with the majority of the remaining visits being for follow-up for a previous illness (14 percent). New illnesses accounted for the majority of visits to both private and public providers. A larger share of visits to public providers (84 percent) is related to new illnesses than to private providers (76 percent). In contrast, follow-up visits represented a much larger share of visits to private providers (15.5 percent) than to public providers (9.6 percent).

Cost of Visits to Private and Public Providers
On average, a visit to a private facility costs more than 2.4 times the cost of a visit to a public provider (table 4.5). Despite this cost difference, visits to private providers remain frequent. For instance, although a visit to a private physician costs more than 3.8 times as much as a visit to a community health center, there are more than 65 percent more visits to physicians than to community health centers. The most expensive visits are to pharmacies without physicians, followed by visits to nurses, private hospitals, and district hospitals. The least expensive visits are to traditional healers, followed by private physicians. Within the public sector, the least expensive visits are to subcenters, followed by basic health centers and community health centers. The computed average cost does not take into account the severity of illnesses.

Wealth, Distance, and Provider Choice
The survey results reveal that wealthier households and those located farther from a facility are more likely to use private providers. Wealthier households are significantly more likely than poor ones to use private pharmacies with physicians. Households living far from a health facility

Table 4.5   Average Cost per Visit and Total Number of Health Care Visits

Provider	Average cost per visit (Af)	Number of visits[a]
All private providers	348	1,205
Physician	339	1,076
Health clinic	136	8
Hospital	562	17
Pharmacy with physician	254	56
Pharmacy without physician	935	25
Midwife	160	5
Nurse	583	6
Mullah	240	10
Traditional healer	50	2
All public providers	144	287
Community health worker	122	5
District hospital	358	65
Subcenter	48	61
Basic health center	81	104
Community health center	89	49
Other	607	3
All visits	308	1,492

Source: Author, based on survey conducted for this book.
Note: Includes user fees, drugs, and so forth but not transportation cost.
a. Figures include only visits for which cost information was available.

are significantly more likely to use a private pharmacy without a physician than households living within two hours of a facility. Results from the Afghanistan Household Survey (Ministry of Public Health 2006) also indicate that wealth is positively correlated with visits to health facilities in general. Although wealthier households' use of private providers may give public providers space to focus on the poor, the fact that remote households also rely on private providers is a source of concern, given the higher cost of private providers.

Antenatal Care and Provider Choice

Demand for pregnancy-related services is equally split between private and public providers (table 4.6).[1] Among private providers, physicians in solo practice account for the largest share (35.6 percent), followed by midwives (12.7 percent). Demand for services from traditional birth attendants is greater than demand for nurses, private hospitals, and private clinics combined. The variations across provinces are large. In Badghis demand for antenatal care is almost entirely for private providers; in Baghlan and Nimroz demand for publicly provided service is slightly higher.

Table 4.6   Provider Used during Most Recent Pregnancy in Four Provinces
(percent of all pregnancy-related services)

Sector/provider	Badghis	Baghlan	Laghman	Nimroz	All four provinces
Private sector	96 (51)	44 (31)	53 (47)	48 (52)	58 (181)
Physician	45.3 (24)	16.9 (12)	47.8 (43)	33.0 (36)	35.6 (115)
Midwife	30.2 (16)	16.9 (12)	0	11.9 (13)	12.7 (41)
Traditional birth attendant	7.5 (4)	4.2 (3)	0	0	2.2 (7)
Hospital	0	0	0	2.8 (3)	0.9 (3)
Health clinic	0	0	1.1 (1)	0	0.3 (1)
Nurse	1.9 (1)	0	0	0	0.3 (1)
Other	11.3 (6)	5.6 (4)	3.3 (3)	0	5.6 (13)
Public sector	4 (2)	56 (39)	47 (41)	52 (57)	42 (139)
Basic health center	0	7.0 (5)	14.4 (13)	41.3 (45)	19.5 (63)
Community health center or community health worker	0	47.9 (34)	0	0	10.5 (34)
District hospital	1.9 (1)	1.4 (1)	12.2 (11)	10.1 (11)	7.4 (24)
Subcenter	1.9 (1)	0 (0)	21.1 (19)	0.9 (1)	6.5 (21)

Source: Author, based on survey conducted for this book.
Note: Number of visits is shown in parentheses. Household survey implementation in Loghar province was stopped after the survey team was threatened. The same week, a team of international NGO personnel were murdered on the road between Puli Allam and Kabul.

Family Planning

Three out of four households prefer private health care providers for information on family planning (demand for family planning is measured here by stated preference rather than actual services used). Although only 26 percent of private providers provide information on family planning and only about 4 percent offer any family planning services, private providers are the preferred source of information on family planning.

Child Immunizations

Public providers are meeting almost all of the demand for immunizations. Public providers administer 92 percent of Bacillus Calmette-Guerin (BCG); 92 percent of oral polio vaccine (OPV); 93 percent of diphtheria, pertussis, and tetanus (DPT); and 94 percent of measles immunizations. In general, it appears that the choice between public and private providers is driven by availability and price rather than by quality of services.

Types and Quality of Service

In this section, the types of services supplied and perceived quality of care are discussed. Availability of services is assessed in terms of both individual services and packages of services.

Types of Services

The private sector mainly provides curative services as well as some maternal and child health services (table 4.7). The most common services include routine physical exams (72 percent of all providers provide this service), diagnostic services and drug prescriptions (67.1 percent), and pharmaceuticals and mental health counseling (30.2 percent). A significant proportion of the private sector (45.9 percent) also provides general health information, including information on family planning. Few private practitioners administer immunizations (7.1 percent) or provide specialized services, such as surgery (19.5 percent), dental care (7.4 percent), or diagnostic X-rays or ultrasound (2.7 percent). In general, there appears to be some overlap of services between the public and private sectors, with a few exceptions, including preventive services, such as immunization, and specialized services, which are provided mainly by the public sector.

Across the surveyed provinces, there are significant differences in the types of services provided by the private sector. In Badghis the availability of all types of curative and specialized services is much lower than average. At the same time, the availability of services related to maternal and child health is highest. Baghlan appears to have the widest range of services. It performs better than average for almost all types of services and has a high proportion of providers who are prepared to diagnose or treat malaria and tuberculosis.

Service availability by type of provider. Among private providers, midwives and traditional birth attendants are the largest suppliers of maternal and child health services (table 4.8).[2] The supply of these services from physicians is limited. Physicians in solo practice being the dominant private providers, they supply most of the other services. Immunization services are supplied primarily by midwives, followed by physicians. Most dental services and drug provision are handled by traditional healers.

Availability of service packages. There are serious gaps in the availability of privately provided primary health care services, both basic and comprehensive (table 4.9). Services are clustered into six groups of related services. These groupings are not necessarily mutually exclusive;

Table 4.7   Percentage of Private Providers Offering Various Types of Health Care in Five Provinces

Service	Badghis	Baghlan	Laghman	Logar	Nimroz	All five provinces
General curative						
Routine physical exam	37.5	86.2	91.7	92.9	92.3	72.0
Diagnosis and prescription of drugs	33.9	82.8	88.9	85.7	80.8	67.1
Provision of drugs	25.5	22.2	38.9	50.0	39.6	30.3
Mental health or counseling services	15.4	14.3	47.2	14.3	57.7	30.2
Maternal and child health						
Healthy family information	30.8	50.0	33.3	55.6	36.4	45.9
Antenatal care	50.2	42.9	25.0	44.4	36.0	41.4
Postnatal care	45.3	39.3	19.4	50.0	32.0	35.8
Delivery of babies	43.4	35.7	16.7	16.7	24.0	31.1
Family planning information	14.3	32.1	30.6	55.6	26.9	25.8
Immunizations	5.4	14.3	2.8	22.2	4.0	7.1
Specialized services						
Surgery	15.1	25.0	30.6	0	11.5	19.5
Laboratory tests	1.9	28.6	16.2	0	3.8	10.7
Dental services	11.5	7.1	5.6	0	3.8	7.4
Diagnostic X-ray or ultrasound for diagnosis	0	10.7	0	0	4.0	2.7
Public health–related services						
Diagnosis or treatment of malaria	15.1	50.0	60.0	42.9	15.4	33.6
Diagnosis or treatment of tuberculosis	7.5	35.7	8.8	14.3	7.7	13.5

Source: Author, based on survey conducted for this book.

they were framed to reflect different types of services that might reasonably be clustered together:

- *Basic primary health services.* This package consists of routine physical examinations, diagnosis, and prescription of medications, together with provision of healthy family information, antenatal care, and postnatal care.

Table 4.8   Percentage of Private Providers Offering Various Types of Health Care Service in Selected Provinces

Service	Physicians in solo practice (n = 86)	Traditional healers and mullahs (n = 14)	Traditional birth attendants (n = 23)	Midwives (n = 7)
General curative				
Routine physical exam	95	50	0	86
Diagnosis and prescription of drugs	92	36	0	71
Mental health or counseling services	41	14	4	14
Provision of drugs	29	29	4	14
Maternal and child health				
Healthy family information	60	21	4	71
Antenatal care	32	7	74	100
Family planning information	30	0	0	29
Postnatal care	28	7	74	100
Delivery of babies	16	0	96	100
Immunizations	6	0	0	14
Specialized services				
Surgery	25	7	0	14
Laboratory tests	13	0	0	0
Dental services	8	14	4	0
Diagnostic X-ray or ultrasound	2	0	0	0
Public health–related services				
Diagnosis or treatment of malaria	51	7	0	0
Diagnosis or treatment of tuberculosis	20	0	0	0

Source: Author, based on survey conducted for this book.

Table 4.9   Availability of Multiservice Packages in Central and Rural Districts
(percentage of all private providers offering package)

Service package	Overall	Central districts	Rural districts
Basic primary health services	15.5	19.5	9.8
Enhanced primary health services	0.7	1.2	—
Basic maternal health services	24.3	21.8	27.9
Enhanced maternal child health specialty services	8.1	9.2	6.6
One-stop prescription and drug service	23.0	16.3	32.3
Key public health services	10.9	14.0	6.6

Source: Author, based on survey conducted for this book.

- *Enhanced primary health services.* This package includes the basic health services package enhanced by additional primary health care services, including family planning, X-rays for diagnosis, and the diagnosis or treatment of tuberculosis and malaria.
- *Basic maternal and child health specialty services.* This is essentially a one-stop package for maternal health that includes antenatal care, delivery, and postnatal care.
- *Enhanced maternal and child health specialty services.* This is an enhanced package of maternal child health services that includes all basic services plus family planning, healthy family information, and immunizations.
- *One-stop prescription and drug service.* These services are provided by practitioners who both diagnose conditions and prescribe and provide the drugs with which to treat them.
- *Key public health services.* These services are provided by practitioners who diagnose or treat tuberculosis and malaria.

Although 15 percent of private providers deliver basic primary services, less than 1 percent provide enhanced primary health services. Almost one in five private providers makes basic maternal and child health services available, but only 8 percent offer enhanced maternal and child health services.

Provider caseload. Private providers vary significantly in their service capacity. Physicians in solo practice have the heaviest caseload capacity (visits per week) and are the most diverse providers in terms of capacity (table 4.10). The second-heaviest caseload is borne by traditional healers.

Quality of Service
Quality of care is assessed here based on a few proxy indicators, including staffing patterns, the level of formal training of staff, facility infrastructure, and perceived quality measures:

- *Staffing.* More than three-quarters of private providers operate without any medical support staff of any kind. The one-quarter that has support staff comprises physicians in solo practice, clinics and hospitals, and pharmacies. About 74 percent of physicians in solo practice who have staff have other physicians, physician assistants, nurses, or midwives. However, 27 percent of these "medical professional" support staff do not have formal credentials.

Table 4.10   Mean Caseload by Type of Private Provider
(number of visits per week)

Provider	Mean caseload
Physician	82.5
(*n* = 78)	(137.6)
Traditional healer	31.3
(*n* = 6)	(45.2)
Pharmacy without physician	19.6
(*n* = 5)	(28.3)
Midwife	16.5
(*n* = 6)	(11.8)
Mullah	7.3
(*n* = 7)	(10.2)
Traditional birth attendant	4.6
(*n* = 11)	(4.8)

Source: Author, based on survey conducted for this book.
Note: Means are not computed for provider types with fewer than five cases.
Figures in parentheses are standard deviations.

A large proportion of private providers (81 percent) have nonprofessional support staff in addition to medical professionals. Two-fifths (41 percent) have administrative staff engaged in greeting or some other form of patient service, and about 30 percent have staff responsible for ordering or maintaining supplies or some other form of logistical support. Very few (14 percent) have staff assigned to medical records management.

- *Formal training.* More than 70 percent of health workers in the private sector have medical training. This includes training in nursing, in work as a physician assistant, in paramedic work, in "training in a related field," and even "two years college in Pakistan"; it does not include a medical degree. The extent of formal training varies by type of provider. Almost all physicians (96 percent) report having formal training that qualifies for a medical degree. Although 83 percent of pharmacy operators have formal training, only 57 percent of midwives do. None of the traditional birth attendants has formal training. The extent of formal training among private providers varies significantly across districts. In the central districts, 82 percent of providers have formal training in their fields. In contrast, in rural districts only 58 percent have such training.

  Few private providers have formal training in public health. Only 29 percent of physicians received training in tuberculosis and Directly

Observed Therapy Short-Course (DOTS), and only 31 percent received training in malaria diagnosis and treatment. One-third of physicians and two-thirds of midwives received recent training in maternal and child health. None of the traditional birth attendants received training in these areas.

- *Facility infrastructure.* None of the private facilities has the basic infrastructure commonly found in public facilities. One in three facilities does not have electricity, and about three in four do not have piped water. Facility infrastructure is likely to have an impact on the quality of service provided and the efficiency with which providers can serve their patients. More than 80 percent of facilities have a telephone connection.

- *Perceived quality.* Consumers rated the services of private providers as comparable to those of public facilities (table 4.11). Additional measures examined patient satisfaction with the quality and outcomes of services. Overall, most visits were rated "adequate" (68 percent) or "excellent/very good" (24 percent). The quality of care at private providers was rated as comparable to that of public providers. Patients' ratings of the outcomes of their visits were also quite positive, with no significant differences between their rating of private and public sector providers.

Hence, although quality in the private sector is low in terms of structural quality measures, including infrastructure and staffing, the perceived quality of care does not differ from that of the public sector.

Table 4.11   Rating of Service Quality of Public and Private Providers
(percentage of survey respondents)

Rating	Total	Private	Public
Positive	24.1 (385)	25.0 (312)	21.2 (73)
Excellent; couldn't be better	4.0 (64)	4.3 (54)	2.9 (10)
Very good, but could be better	20.1 (321)	20.7 (258)	18.2 (63)
Adequate	68.2 (1,087)	67.7 (845)	69.7 (242)
Negative	7.4 (118)	7.0 (88)	8.6 (30)
Not very good	5.6 (89)	5.2 (65)	6.9 (24)
Terrible	1.8 (29)	1.8 (23)	1.7 (6)
Undetermined	0.3 (5)	0.2 (3)	0.6 (2)
Total	100 (1,595)	100 (1,248)	100 (347)

Source: Author, based on survey conducted for this book.
Note: Figures in parentheses indicate number of providers.

Constraints and Future Outlook

This section describes the constraints the private sector faces. It examines the process of starting a private health care practice, reports on private providers' business outlook, and identifies constraints on operation and possible expansion.

Starting a Private Health Care Practice

In general, starting a private business in health services is a relatively easy process. About 43 percent of those surveyed found it not difficult at all to start a practice. Only one in five reported that starting a practice had been difficult. Providers without formal training were slightly more likely to encounter difficulty starting their practice.[3]

About 50 percent of start-up capital was obtained through the provider's own savings or funds raised through freelance medical practices (table 4.12). This figure partly reflects the low level of development of the credit market in rural Afghanistan. The data do not show the exact amount of financing obtained from each of these sources, but they do indicate in broad terms whether the amount constitutes the primary source or a large or small part of the start-up capital. No single source emerges as the most significant source of financing. In a positive sign of the emergence of a credit market, microfinance programs provided the start-up capital for some, albeit a small proportion of, private providers.

Providers with formal training were substantially more likely than providers without formal training to have relied on fees or their own savings. Sixty percent of providers with formal training identified fees and

Table 4.12   Sources of Start-Up Capital
(percentage of survey respondents)

Importance of support	Fees	Personal social networks		Community social networks		Microfinance or local NGOs
		Own savings	Relatives or friends	Village leaders or shura	Other providers	
Provided most of the support	15	23	5	2	1	0
Provided a large amount but not primary source	30	21	9	8	7	4
Provided a small amount of help	19	32	30	17	12	12

Source: Author, based on survey conducted for this book.

50 percent identified their own savings as sources of their start-up capital. In contrast, for providers without formal training, the corresponding figures were 13 percent from fees and 30 percent from own savings.

Private Providers' Business Outlook

Two in three providers believe that their operation is successful and would like to expand it. A large number of providers would like to either expand the range of services they are providing (83 percent) or expand geographically (69 percent). In terms of future prospects, 60 percent of providers see themselves doing the same work in 5 years' time and 55 percent see themselves doing the same work in 10 years' time.

Constraints on Operation and Possible Expansion

Among the constraints providers face, the lack of qualified health workers emerged at the top of the list. An attempt was made to measure the level of constraints private providers would face either in continuing or expanding their current practices. Recruiting and retaining qualified health workers was cited as the major constraint by 28 percent of providers. The second-most-cited constraint was infrastructure, identified by 24 percent. Infrastructure constraints are not surprising given the small number of facilities that have sources of water and regular electricity. Access to credit, especially to meet operating costs, was the third-most important constraint. In contrast to public facilities, private providers exhibit little concern over security (4 percent).

In summary, although setting up private health care services is not perceived as difficult, mobilizing start-up capital is challenging. Most private providers have to resort to their own savings or the help of relatives to mobilize the necessary resources. Despite difficulty in mobilizing the resources to enter the market and stay operational, most private providers would like to expand their practices either geographically or in terms of service. As in the public sector, recruiting and maintaining trained health workers is a major constraint limiting expansion.

Concluding Remarks: Findings and Recommendations

The fact that the majority of health services are provided by the private sector makes the stewardship role of the MOPH essential. The complementary nature of the services of the private sector can be expanded through policies that harness the sector's energy. Although the private sector provides mainly complementary services, it has also demonstrated its potential to contribute to activities that are traditionally left to the public sector. For instance, private providers are active in information, education and communication/behavior change communication (IEC/BCC) activities, and they are the preferred source of information for family planning. Investments to prepare them to be more effective health promoters and to motivate them to become more consistent and proactive agents of change are worth exploring. Working in parallel with national media health campaigns, private providers could be used to convey key health messages.

The ongoing effort to establish a unit within the MOPH to work with the private sector is a step in the right direction. The MOPH has begun preparing related documents and establishing a new unit, including a task force for organizing private sector–related activities, which are scattered across different departments. The urgency of acting on this front has been recognized. This volume should help guide the initial stages of the unit's engagement with the private sector.

Quality assurance is an area on which the MOPH needs to focus in the short term. Parallel to efforts to improve the quality of care of publicly provided health services, the ministry should work to improve the quality of service in the private sector. This can be done by encouraging the participation of private providers in quality assessment surveys along the lines of the Balanced Score Card.

Various means can be used to encourage the participation of private providers in quality assessments, including regulatory measures, contracting, and incentives. The MOPH has the full range of regulatory instruments at its disposal to work with the private sector:

- *Regulatory controls and restrictions*. Regulatory instruments involve legal requirements to which providers must conform. Violating these restrictions would result in some kind of penalty.
- *Incentives*. Incentives are bonus payments and penalties that the ministry would develop to encourage providers to change behavior in order to achieve desired targets for quality or coverage.
- *Contracting*. The MOPH could exert significant influence over the private sector by contracting with private providers for complementary services or expansion of some services in the BPHS.
- *Information dissemination*. Information dissemination involves making information on providers available to users so that consumers can make informed decisions that encourage providers to improve service quality.

These instruments are not necessarily mutually exclusive and would perhaps work best if the MOPH used them in combination.

Large-scale implementation of mandatory participation in quality assessments is not currently viable. Under the mandatory approach, the MOPH would define a minimum acceptable level of quality and assess facilities to determine compliance. This approach would be highly demanding in the breadth and depth of information it would require to implement, and enforcing compliance would be costly and prone to capture. The current inclination of the MOPH, nevertheless, is toward using such a regulatory instrument. The ministry needs to examine its ability to rely exclusively on this instrument. Enforcement capacity, in particular, is a major challenge. However, the ministry could use this instrument for licensing, if not for regular monitoring.

Using incentives is an option the MOPH should explore to improve quality of care. To create incentives for increasing quality, it could make the accreditation of facilities conditional on their attaining a certain standard. Private providers could be encouraged to participate in quality assessments to demonstrate their service quality and then be accredited accordingly. The demand for accreditation would increase if the ministry supplemented the accreditation process by disseminating information on the service quality of private providers to the public and selectively contracting with private providers that become accredited.

Notes

1. Among all households, 14.2 percent reported that health facilities were too far to visit, 11.1 percent reported there was no need to visit health facilities for antenatal care, and 7.1 percent reported that visits were too expensive.

2. The small number of providers of other types (nurses, private hospitals, private clinics) did not allow meaningful analysis of service profiles for these groups.

3. The sample is not large enough to discern whether there are significant differences among types of providers.

CHAPTER 5

Human Resources for Health

This chapter focuses on human resources working in the public sector and working for providers financed by the public sector through contracts. The data used in this chapter are not exhaustive.[1] They should be viewed as providing a lower-bound estimate of the total health worker pool in the country, for two reasons: the database contains information only on Afghan health workers (foreign nationals are not recorded) and health workers in the for-profit private sector are not taken into account.

Despite significant progress since 2003 (1382 AC) in addressing human resource constraints, the labor force in the health sector continues to face critical challenges. Notable progress has been made in the training and deployment of community midwives and community health workers (CHWs). Despite these efforts, however, the health sector workforce continues to face problems that can be summarized as three major imbalances:

- *Geographic imbalance.* A disproportionately large number of health care workers are concentrated in cities and periurban areas while rural areas still suffer from shortages.
- *Gender imbalance.* There is still a shortage of female staff, especially in rural areas.

- *Skills-mix imbalance*. There is a shortage of staff with public health, reproductive health, and child health skills.

An additional problem is the vacancy rate for health workers within the Ministry of Public Health (MOPH). Ministry records show that about 40 percent of the total workforce, which translates to 7,411 people, are employed by the MOPH as civil servants. The approved staffing of the MOPH is 14,002 positions; the Ministry of Finance's records show 11,291 individuals employed by the MOPH. Depending on which figure is taken as the expected number of staff of the MOPH, the vacancy rate is 19–34 percent.

Such a high vacancy rate offers an opportunity for the MOPH to address its human resource imbalances. In filling the vacant positions, the MOPH can focus on hiring a disproportionate share of female health workers, filling positions in remote areas, and focusing on health workers in the skill areas in which there are current shortages.

Although the human resources problem is common knowledge, there is little information on the extent of the problem to guide policy formulation. This chapter describes the level, structure, and distribution of the health care workforce in Afghanistan and discusses policy options for addressing current imbalances. Policy alternatives derived from experience within and outside Afghanistan regarding hiring, retaining, and redistributing existing and incoming human resources for health are discussed in this chapter.

The remainder of the chapter is structured as follows. The next section presents the structure of existing human resources. The following section estimates the demand for health workers. The last section presents concluding remarks.

Level and Structure of Human Resources for Health

This section examines several aspects of human resources for health in Afghanistan. It describes the deployment of current human resources, the distribution by function, the geographic distribution, and the skill mix of health workers by type of facility.

Deployment of Current Human Resources

There are nearly 20,000 registered health workers in Afghanistan, 40 percent employed by the MOPH and 60 percent by NGOs. Of the MOPH staff, most positions are at MOPH headquarters and provincial offices; less than 5 percent of staff work at Ministry of Public Health–Strengthening Mechanism (MOPH–SM) facilities (table 5.1). Among NGO staff, four NGOs—Badakshan Development Network (BDN), Ibn Sina, Care of Afghan Families (CAF), and the Swedish Committee for Afghanistan (SCA)—employ about 20 percent of the total health workforce.

Table 5.1   Number and Percentage Share of Health Care Staff, by Institution, 2008 (1387 AC)

Institution	Number registered	Percentage of total health care workforce
Ministry of Public Health and Ministry of Higher Education	7,411	40.3
Ministry of Public Health (headquarters and provincial offices)	6,652	36.2
Ministry of Public Health–Strengthening Mechanism	753	4.1
Ministry of Higher Education	6	–
Contracted nongovernmental organizations (NGOs)	10,993	59.7
Badakshan Development Network (BDN)	1,203	6.5
Ibn Sina	974	5.3
Care of Afghan Families (CAF)	779	4.2
Swedish Committee for Afghanistan (SCA)	737	4.0
International Medical Corps (IMC)	727	4.0
Coordination of Humanitarian Assistance (CHA)	627	3.4
MOVE	546	3.0
STEP Health & Development Organization	533	2.9
BRAC Afghanistan Bank	522	2.8
Aide Médicale Internationale (AMI)	462	2.5
Health Net (TPO)	346	1.9
Loma Linda University (LLU)	339	1.8
Afghan Health & Development Services (AHDS)	305	1.7
Norwegian Afghanistan Committee (NAC)	285	1.5
Aga Khan Development Network (AKDN)	244	1.3
Sanayee Development Foundation (SDF)	218	1.2
Medical Refresher Courses for Afghans (MRCA)	206	1.1
Merlin	199	1.1
Adventist Development and Relief Agency (ADRA)	196	1.1
Agency for Assistance and Development of Afghanistan (AADA)	184	1.0
International Assistance Mission (IAM)	169	0.9
International Committee of the Red Cross (ICRC)	141	0.8
Japanese Cooperation (TODAI)	117	0.6
Social & Health Development Program (SHDP)	116	0.6

(continued)

Table 5.1   *(continued)*

Institution	Number registered	Percentage of total health care workforce
Save the Children	112	0.6
Solidarity for Afghan Families (SAF)	110	0.6
World Vision International (WVI)	86	0.5
Provincial Reconstruction Teams (PRT)	82	0.4
Afghan Red Crescent Society (ARCS)	61	0.3
Italian Cooperation	45	0.2
Jahanita	35	0.2
Afghan Institute of Learning	33	0.2
Médecins du Monde	30	0.2
Medair	23	0.1
SHUHADA	19	0.1
Management Systems International (MSI)	16	0.1
JACK	13	0.1
CWS	12	0.1
SOZO International	10	0.1
Other	82	0.4
14 institutions with fewer than 10 Afghans listed in database	49	0.3
NGO subtotal	10,993	59.7
Total	18,404	100

Source: Human resources database (Ministry of Public Health 2008b [1387 AC]).
Note: – = Negligible.

NGOs employ 9 out of 10 health workers in facilities providing the basic package of health services (BPHS) (subcenters, basic health centers, comprehensive health centers, and district hospitals). Among staff employed in BPHS facilities, NGOs employ 88–95 percent of physicians, midwives, nurses, allied health professionals, technicians, and outreach workers, and MOPH–SM facilities employ 3–6 percent. The MOPH and NGOs employ about equal numbers of health workers at provincial hospitals. At the specialist hospital level, the MOPH is virtually the sole employer.

The level of staffing of BPHS facilities appears to satisfy BPHS requirements. On average, basic health centers are staffed by 4.7 health workers, comprehensive centers have 11.7 health workers, district hospitals have 23.2 staff, and provincial hospitals have 58.0 staff. The number of health workers in the largest institutions can be as high as 180.4.

Health workers are concentrated in regional/specialty hospitals. The number of health workers in such hospitals (staffed by MOPH employees) is greater than the total number working in basic health centers and district hospitals combined (largely NGO staff) (figure 5.1). A significant number of staff work in health facilities that have not been identified by type.

Movement of health workers among providers is limited: slightly more than 1 percent of health workers changed employers between 2007/08 and 2008/09 (1386–87 AC). Almost all movements observed were in Kabul and its surroundings. Movement between providers is highly discouraged as a matter of policy. A national salary policy was formulated to minimize competition among providers and reduce the movement of health workers.

Movement is greater within the MOPH workforce. Over the same period, about 10 percent of the MOPH workforce, of which 85 percent are highly skilled technicians and specialists, moved to other institutions. Data on these movements started to be recorded only recently, so historical trends are unknown. Movements to and from the MOPH are thought to have been common in the early years of the ministry and during the time NGOs were starting to establish themselves. Most of those movements were not captured.

Figure 5.1   Number of Staff Working for NGOs and the Ministry of Public Health, by Type of Facility

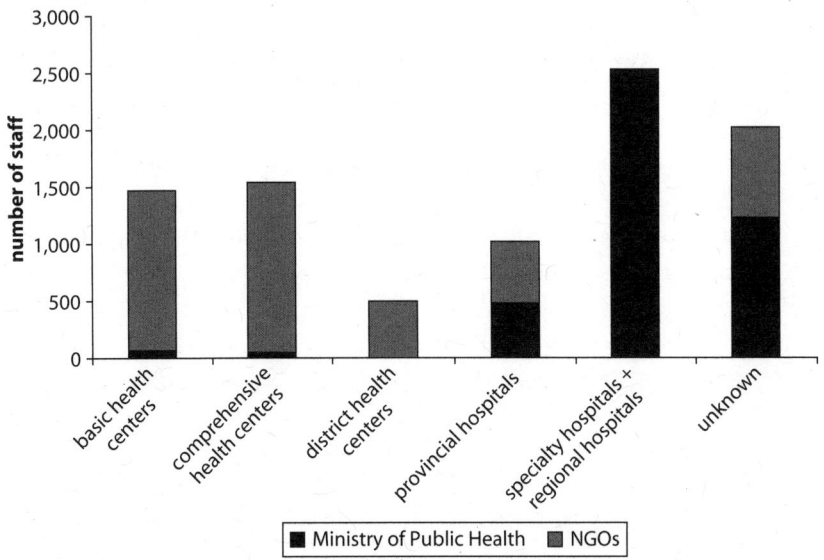

Source: Human resources database (Ministry of Public Health 2008b [1387 AC]).

Distribution by Function

The composition of the workforce reveals that 45 percent are physicians, midwives, and nurses; 23 percent are allied health professionals and technicians; and 30 percent are support staff (table 5.2)[2] Physicians and nurses are proportionately distributed between the MOPH and NGOs that are managing mainly primary care facilities. In contrast, midwives and allied staff are highly concentrated among NGOs. The share of staff working in management is skewed toward the MOPH, with 88 percent of management staff working at the ministry.

The number of outreach workers in the database is grossly underestimated. Most outreach workers are CHWs operating voluntarily. These workers are compensated by their communities or by directly charging patients a fee for services. They do not directly report to the MOPH and do not show up in the database.

Preliminary assessments show that the number of CHWs is much higher than captured by MOPH data. Although there are no comprehensive data documenting the number and status of CHWs in all provinces, a number of attempts have been made to build data on active CHWs in the country. According to the data collected by the Community-Based Health Care Task Force of the MOPH, there were 14,136 active CHWs in 2006/07 (1385 AC) (MOPH, JHU, and IIHMR 2007a), more than half of them female. Recent data on the deployment of CHWs in 13 of Afghanistan's 34 provinces show that 8,386 CHWs were actively operating as of June 2008 (1387 AC). Another study shows a total of 18,000 CHWs distributed in the entire country. Although the actual number of CHWs operating is not clear, the total number is likely to be high and include a large share of women.

Table 5.2   Percentage of Staff in Different Job Categories, by Employer, 2008 (1387 AC)

Profession	Total	MOPH	MOPH–SM	NGOs
Physicians	21.4	52	2	46
Nurses	16.2	43	3	54
Midwives	7.4	36	3	61
Allied professional and technical support and others	48.6	26	4	71
Outreach	3.9	9	4	87
Management	2.5	88	5	7
Total	100.0	36.7	4.1	59.7

Source: Human resources database (Ministry of Public Health 2008b [1387 AC]).
Note: MOPH = Ministry of Public Health; MOPH–SM = Ministry of Public Health–Strengthening Mechanism; NGOs = nongovernmental organizations.

Geographic Distribution

There are large disparities across provinces in per capita total staff and skill mix. The number of health workers per population ranges from 0.16 in Uruzgan to 1.65 in Kabul (table 5.3). Kabul ranks first in total number of health workers per capita, followed by Nuristan, Jawzian, Paktya, Bamyan, and Panjshir. Not surprisingly, this pattern closely traces the distribution of facilities across provinces. In terms of skill mix, the two provinces that are mainly rural, Panjshir and Nuristan, have the lowest percentages of frontline workers and the highest percentages of support staff. Uruzgan, followed by Samangan and Wardak, has the largest proportion of frontline workers and the lowest proportion of support staff. Balkh, one of the largest provinces, has the lowest percentage (14.8 percent) of allied professional and technical staff. Kabul province has the second-lowest share (15.0 percent) of these positions. The high concentration of the private sector in Balkh and Kabul provinces could explain this pattern.

Female health workers constitute 24 percent of the health workforce, with significant variations across provinces (see table 5.3). In provinces that account for one-third of the population, the proportion of women in the total workforce is higher than the national average. The difference between the highest-ranked and the lowest-ranked province is roughly 23 percentage points. It is not clear what explains these differences. Although insecurity was identified as one of the challenges in recruiting and retaining female health workers, the share of female health workers does not appear to be related to differences in security. For instance, in a relatively secure province (Panjshir), only 10 percent of the health workforce is female, whereas a relatively insecure province (Ghazni) has nearly twice the share of female health workers.

Skill Mix of Health Workers by Type of Facility

Although the level of staffing of BPHS facilities is adequate, the distribution of the skill mix could be improved. There are an average of 4.7 health workers at basic health centers, 11.7 at comprehensive centers, and 23.2 at district hospitals, which appears to be adequate. However, the composition of health workers in basic health centers, comprehensive health centers, and district hospitals shows some imbalances in the distribution of key staff positions, particularly midwives, nurses, and specialists (figure 5.2).

Table 5.3 Staff Allocation by Province, 2008 (1387 AC)

Province	Population (thousands)	Percentage of population that is rural	Percentage of staff in database in June (excluding outreach workers)				Total number of health workers in database	Number of health workers/thousand people	Percentage of health workers who are female
			Management	Frontline	Allied and tech	Support			
Kabul	3,335.0	17.6	3.2	48.6	15.0	33.3	5,518	1.65	31
Herat	1,611.2	73.6	4.3	50.7	24.9	20.1	606	0.38	22
Nangarhar	1,309.4	86.1	0.4	58.3	24.4	16.9	856	0.65	14
Balkh	1,122.6	65.1	0.7	64.4	14.8	20.1	851	0.76	31
Ghazni	1,073.7	95.3	3.6	39.5	28.8	28.2	816	0.76	20
Kandahar	1,037.1	66.9	3.9	59.7	26.9	9.6	387	0.37	21
Faryab	868.8	88.3	3.5	46.9	29.5	20.0	454	0.52	25
Kunduz	866.7	76.1	1.3	57.6	34.3	6.7	297	0.34	20
Takhar	855.5	87.4	4.5	38.8	28.1	28.6	707	0.83	18
Badakshan	831.2	96.2	1.5	41.7	30.4	26.4	542	0.65	25
Helmand	807.5	94.3	0.4	61.7	30.2	7.7	235	0.29	18
Baghlan	789.5	80.5	1.5	51.8	32.6	14.1	469	0.59	23
Ghor	604.4	99.0	3.4	36.5	35.6	24.5	208	0.34	13
Parwan	579.3	91.5	3.9	48.1	30.9	17.2	233	0.40	14
Wardak	522.2	99.5	0.8	57.1	37.9	4.2	240	0.46	16
Khost	502.7	98.1	1.4	46.5	27.2	24.9	346	0.69	13
Sari Pul	488.2	92.5	0.6	60.2	28.2	11.0	181	0.37	23
Paktya	482.4	95.7	1.7	43.2	25.8	29.2	472	0.98	16

Province									
Jawzjan	468.0	79.3	4.0	51.4	17.9	26.6	496	1.06	27
Farah	448.8	93.0	1.7	61.5	26.9	10.0	301	0.67	22
Badghis	433.8	97.1	0.8	47.1	40.8	11.3	240	0.55	11
Daykundi	403.3	99.2	0.0	51.1	38.6	10.2	88	0.22	28
Kunar	394.1	97.1	0.0	55.7	38.8	5.5	183	0.46	13
Bamyan	391.1	97.3	6.0	47.7	32.3	14.0	365	0.93	26
Laghman	390.1	98.9	0.0	63.3	28.9	7.8	270	0.69	12
Kapisa	386.3	99.7	3.0	52.0	33.7	11.4	202	0.52	15
Pakyika	380.7	99.4	7.7	40.1	26.5	25.8	287	0.75	12
Logar	342.9	97.6	0.0	51.7	33.6	14.7	211	0.62	13
Samangan	338.3	92.7	1.8	60.7	32.7	4.8	168	0.50	23
Uruzgan	306.6	97.2	2.0	72.0	22.0	4.0	50	0.16	13
Zabul	265.8	96.2	0.8	48.4	18.9	32.0	122	0.46	11
Nimroz	137.4	83.9	0.0	57.8	35.6	6.7	45	0.33	24
Panjsher	134.4	100.0	1.8	35.1	22.5	40.5	111	0.83	10
Nuristan	129.6	100.0	0.6	35.5	25.8	38.1	155	1.20	8
Total	23,038.6	77.6	2.6	50.0	23.5	23.9	16,712	0.73	24

Source: Human resources database (Ministry of Public Health 2008b [1387 AC]).
Note: Figures exclude workers at community health centers.

Figure 5.2   Distribution of Health Care Workers by Category and Facility Type, 2008 (1387 AC)

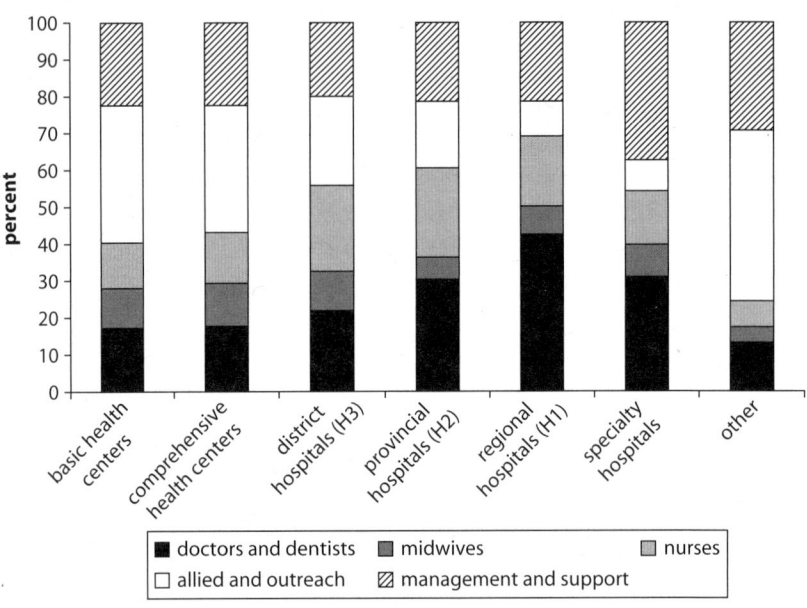

Source: Human resources database (Ministry of Public Health 2008b [1387 AC]).

The share of midwives in larger hospitals (provincial, regional, and specialty) is low. Although the emphasis on increasing the supply of midwives would appear to have been successful measured against the standards set by the BPHS and the essential package of hospital services (EPHS), the larger hospitals appear to be lagging.

The overall mix of physicians and nurses is out of balance, with three physicians for every two nurses. The proportion of nurses in BPHS facilities is higher than in higher-level hospitals. Less than a quarter of the workforce at each of these types of facilities is made up of nurses.

The proportion of physicians in regional and specialist hospitals is particularly high. In all regional hospitals, the proportion of physicians is higher than that of nurses, midwives, allied professionals, and technical support combined. This seems to be an out-of-balance skill mix. The equivalent numbers in specialized hospitals are almost the same (1,217 versus 1,223). This is not an efficient use of the human resources budget. Such large proportions of physicians mean that they cannot be adequately supported by other professionals and place a heavy burden on the budgets of the facilities.

Demand for and Quality of Human Resources

This section begins by examining the human resource requirements needed to meet BPHS and EPHS requirements and Afghanistan's health and nutrition sector strategy goals. It then assesses the quality of the workforce.

Human Resource Requirements

This section provides estimates of the demand for health workers in Afghanistan. Although the private sector contributes significantly to the provision of health services, estimates can be made only for the public sector. It is not possible to estimate the human resource requirement of the private sector because there is not enough information available and most private sector practitioners are also public sector employees.

Therefore, the estimates provided here should be regarded as lower-bound estimates, for two reasons: with the expansion of the private sector, the demand for full-time employees will increase, and the human resource requirements for the public sector are estimated using the staffing requirements of the BPHS and EPHS. Thus, a number of programs with their own demands for health workers are not captured by the staffing needs to deliver these two packages.

Staff needed to meet BPHS and EPHS requirements. Demand estimates are based on the recommended levels of staffing required to deliver the BPHS and EPHS.[3] The estimates do not include facilities that were not part of the BPHS before the revision or the EPHS. The BPHS and EPHS documents specify the staffing requirements for the various types of facilities (table 5.4). As a result of concerns about the initial BPHS and EPHS staffing requirements and subsequent efforts to revise them, the suggested levels are used as guidelines for estimating the demand for various types of health workers.

Overall, the health worker shortage is very severe, with an estimated shortage of 39 percent (table 5.5). On the one hand, meeting the current BPHS and EPHS norms requires a large supply of health workers in all categories except dentists. On the other hand, there are a few health worker categories that are not included in the packages but seem able to fill important gaps in the health worker shortage, including assistant midwives and nurses. It is therefore important to take the BPHS/EPHS requirements as guidelines rather than as rigid rules. For instance, the fact that the BPHS/EPHS standards do not include "assistants"

Table 5.4 **Suggested Frontline Requirements per Facility under the BPHS and EPHS**

	BPHS			BPHS/ EPHS	EPHS	
Profession	Subcenter	Basic health center	Comprehensive health center	District hospital	Provincial hospital	Regional and specialty hospitals
Surgeons, anesthetists, and other specialists	0	0	0	7	17	35
Dentists	0	0	0	0	1	3
Physicians	0	0	2	3	13	28
Feldshers[a]	0	0	0	0	0	0
Midwives	0	0	0	4	9	15
Assistant midwives	0	0	0	0	0	0
Community midwives	0	1	0	0	0	0
Nurses, male	0	1	1	7.5	20	43.5
Nurses, female	0	0	1	7.5	20	43.5
Total frontline health care providers	0	2	4	29	80	168
Number of facilities	176	760	372	57	30	26

Source: Human resources database (Ministry of Public Health 2008b [1387 AC]).

Note: BPHS = basic package of health services; EPHS = essential package of hospital services.
a. A feldsher is an assistant physician trained under the Russian system.

Table 5.5   Total Estimated Requirements for Frontline Health Care Jobs

Profession	Staff required	Existing staff	Shortfall/surplus (percent)
Surgeons, anesthetists, and other specialists	1,819	1,547	−15.0
Dentists	108	194	79.6
Physicians	2,169	1,975	−8.9
Midwives	1,249	1,189	−4.8
Community midwives	760	340	−55.3
Nurses, male	3,359	2,140	−36.3
Nurses, female	2,599	378	−85.5
Feldshers/assistant physicians	n.a.	527	n.a.
Assistant midwives	n.a.	97	n.a.
Anesthesia nurses and skilled workers	n.a.	178	n.a.
Assistant nurses, male	n.a.	101	n.a.
Assistant nurses, female	n.a.	25	n.a.
Total	12,063	8,691	−38.8

Source: Human resources database (Ministry of Public Health 2008b [1387 AC]).
Note: Requirements cover all facilities, including drug addiction centers, maternal and child clinics, and tuberculosis clinics. Outreach workers are not included. n.a. = Not available.

should not be interpreted to mean that assistants cannot or should not be deployed. Building in flexibility so that existing health workers are deployed and fully utilized is critical to addressing shortages in some areas. Given the existing mix of health workers, there should be the opportunity to allow, for instance, physicians at BPHS facilities to fill nurse or midwife vacancies.

Staff needed to meet health and nutrition sector strategy goals. Conservative estimates of the human resource requirements for attaining the health and nutrition sector strategy (HNSS) goals show a shortfall of 43.1 percent. The HNSS stipulates that the government intends to expand coverage of the BPHS from its 2008/09 (1387 AC) level of 62–90 percent. Assuming that the current proportion of BPHS facilities is maintained and no district hospitals need to be built to achieve the HNSS coverage, it is estimated that a significant number of new facilities will be needed, with corresponding increases in staff (tables 5.6 and 5.7).

Quality of the Workforce
The HNSS identified the quality of the health workforce as a problem. According to the HNSS, ad hoc training meant to respond to the state of

Table 5.6   Estimated Number of Additional Facilities Needed to Meet the Health and Nutrition Sector Strategy Coverage Target

Item	Subcenters	Basic health centers	Comprehensive health centers
Number of facilities, 2008/09 (1387 AC)	176	760	372
Proportion of total facilities (percent)	13.5	58.1	28.4
Estimated additional facilities needed	7	124	30

Source: Author's estimates, based on data from the Health Management Information System (Ministry of Public Health).

Table 5.7   Estimated Number of Health Workers Required to Meet the Health and Nutrition Sector Strategy Coverage Target

Profession	Subcenters	Basic health centers	Comprehensive health centers
Surgeons, anesthetists, and other specialists	0	0	0
Dentists	0	0	0
Physicians	0	0	60
Feldshers	0	0	0
Midwives	7	0	0
Assistant midwives	0	0	0
Community midwives	0	124	0
Nurses, male	7	124	30
Nurses, female	0	0	30
Total	13	247	118
Number of additional facilities	7	124	30

Source: Author's estimates, based on data from the Health Management Information System (Ministry of Public Health).
Note: A feldsher is an assistant physician trained under the Russian system.

emergency has resulted in health workers who are working beyond their capacities. Review of the private sector also reveals the urgency and significance of improving the quality of health workers (see chapter 4). Moreover, according to data from the Balanced Scorecard, knowledge among health providers has either stagnated or started to decline.

Training of health workers in Afghanistan is highly heterogeneous. It could benefit from some standardization and accreditation of training institutions. Accreditation of training institutions ensures that the training delivered meets specified standards. It can improve the quality of health worker training and thus the quality of the workforce. This is particularly important for physicians, who receive training from many different types of institutions and even different countries. For historical reasons, the level and quality of training of midwives and nurses have also been heterogeneous. Recent developments in providing uniform training for community midwives and subsequent accreditation are a step forward.

Until professional councils are in place, it is necessary for the MOPH to continue to conduct health worker registration and accredit curricula and courses in collaboration with the Ministry of Higher Education.[4] This task will be taken over by professional councils when they are established for each discipline and for the general Health Professions Council. The councils' tasks are planned to include further developing and maintaining a health care worker registration system for national and overseas applicants; accrediting training institutes and curricula and ensuring adherence to standards; and developing standards, in collaboration with the Ministry of Higher Education.

Given that the private sector provides about two-thirds of curative health services, health worker registration and accreditation efforts need to include private providers. Although there are ongoing efforts to facilitate accreditation of private facilities,[5] they cover only a minor part of the private sector. A significant part of the private sector is made up of individual practitioners who practice out of small facilities in rural areas. Accrediting this group would be an enormous task for the MOPH; certifying training programs in critical areas would be one option. There is already some experience with this approach, such as a training program for pharmacies provided by an NGO, that could be expanded. The training certificate displayed in these pharmacies serves as an indication to consumers of potentially higher-quality service. Other options for improving quality among private providers are discussed in chapter 4.

Concluding Remarks: Findings and Recommendations

The current draft of Afghanistan's human resources policy may need to be revised to better reflect a strategic vision and implementation approach. The human resources for health strategy and policy need to translate the guiding principles into a coherent action plan for addressing human resource issues in the country. The action plan should specify the responsibilities of various actors, the resource requirements, and the timeframe for implementation. In the short term, training community midwives and nurses must form the cornerstone of such a plan.

Incentives

The government should create incentives to make working in the health sector more attractive for women and people willing to work in remote areas. The government retains near monopoly power over the medical education system; it could, for example, grant preferential admission to women and people committing to work in remote areas. It is also possible to make postings to attractive locations conditional on first fulfilling a commitment to work in a remote area. This approach is used in Bangladesh, where points are awarded for working in remote areas and accumulation of points increases the likelihood of future postings in more attractive locations.

Professional development opportunities for health workers working outside Kabul should be expanded. The data show that health workers are unlikely to find opportunities for professional development once they leave Kabul. Making professional development opportunities available in more remote areas may provide incentives for working in these locations.

Payments and benefits that are related to place of work and performance could also be piloted. A proposed experiment, through the results-based financing pilot, to motivate health workers through additional payment linked to performance would provide new sets of evidence on the possibility of using such a mechanism to recruit and retain workers in remote areas.

Other Alternatives

The MOPH could pilot hiring health facility staff on a contract basis. Doing so is useful for a number of reasons:

- It would help the MOPH avoid any long-term contingent liabilities that hiring permanent employees would imply. Given that the current budget share for staff salary and benefits is about 50 percent, this could be an attractive alternative to the ministry.
- It would increase managers' ability to ensure that staff focus on performance.
- It would allow flexible remuneration, which in turn would be a useful instrument for promptly responding to emerging human resource problems. Contractual hiring could also be a broader intervention to attract and retain female health workers in remote areas than interventions involving salary increases.

All of these options should be piloted and evaluated as part of the workforce planning process before implementing them on a larger scale.

Notes

1. The analysis relies heavily on the database developed by the ministry. This database is still a work in progress and does not contain all the human resources available in the country. However, it contains sufficient information to satisfy the needs for human resource information at all levels within the ministry. As of late August 2008 (1387 AC), there were 18,404 individuals in this database.

2. Detailed descriptions of each of these categories and the numbers in the workforce are indicated in appendix F.

3. Initial BPHS documents do not include staffing requirements for subcenters, because they were not part of BPHS facilities during the early stages. Subcenters are the products of innovation by the implementing NGOs in response to the difficult geography and terrain of rural Afghanistan. In practice, each of these facilities is staffed with a nurse and a midwife. Moreover, about 68 facilities were not included in either the BPHS or the EPHS, including maternal and child health clinics, drug addiction centers, and tuberculosis clinics (see appendix F). Assuming that each of the 68 facilities not included in either package would require two physicians and two nurses, there will be an additional requirement for 136 physicians, 68 male nurses, and 68 female nurses. These assumptions, added to the EPHS and BPHS staffing patterns, would result in the national requirements for these frontline health providers.

4. Professional councils are being established in Afghanistan to move toward self-regulation of medical professions. To date, a midwifery council has been established, and the process to establish councils for nursing and pharmacy is under way. Having independent professional councils would separate accreditation from training. Such councils would register professionals, accredit institutions and curricula, and arbitrate cases of professional misconduct.

5. The strategic planning retreat held by the MOPH and its partners in November 2007 (1386 AC) stressed the need to regulate the quality of private providers.

CHAPTER 6

Strengthening the Basic Package of Health Services

The basic package of health services (BPHS) is widely viewed as central to the success the Ministry of Public Health (MOPH) has achieved in improving health services and health outcomes in Afghanistan. The BPHS is essentially a strategy for delivering key primary health care interventions to rural areas of the country. It comprises a set of prioritized, high-impact, cost-effective interventions; a specific service delivery structure that includes community health workers (CHWs) in health posts at basic health centers, comprehensive health centers, district hospitals, and most recently, health subcenters and mobile units; and a series of standards or norms that apply to services, staffing, equipment, and supplies in each of the different types of facilities.

The BPHS has been critical in ensuring that all stakeholders working in the health sector in Afghanistan focus on a common strategy established by the MOPH. As such, it has been central to establishing and maintaining the stewardship role of the MOPH. The BPHS has also developed wide "brand recognition," which has made it shorthand for a series of policies and strategies that focus on delivering high-impact primary health care interventions, ensuring that adequate resources and effort are dedicated to improving the coverage of services to the large rural population and to preventing excessive capture of scarce public funds by urban elites, improving equity in access to services and maintaining a focus on the poor, and promoting careful monitoring and evaluation (M&E). The interventions included in the BPHS are widely credited with being the major driver of reductions in the infant and under-five mortality rates described in chapter 2.

The BPHS has evolved since 2002 (1381 AC), when consensus was reached to focus limited resources on key health interventions. In 2002, as part of a series of two joint donor missions, there was broad agreement that the government was going to have to focus on a package of services rather than try to do everything. With assistance from the World Health Organization and the U.S. Agency for International Development (USAID), the MOPH developed a draft, which was widely discussed and published in 2003 (1382 AC). A revision of the BPHS was published in 2005, and a further revised version is expected to be available in 2010 (1388 AC).

The BPHS focuses on high-impact primary health care interventions, such as child immunization (through routine services as well as mass vaccination campaigns against measles, neonatal tetanus, and polio); micronutrient supplementation and nutrition screening; tuberculosis and malaria control; antenatal, obstetrical, and postpartum care; family planning; and basic curative services, including integrated management of childhood illnesses (IMCI). The version of the BPHS that was updated in 2005 (1384 AC) added activities related to mental health and disability.

In addition to defining priority interventions, the BPHS specifies the organization of primary health care services. The organization of services is based on a somewhat hierarchical network of health facilities, including district hospitals (serving areas with populations of 100,000–300,000), comprehensive health centers (serving areas with populations of 30,000–60,000), basic health centers (serving areas with populations of 15,000–30,000), and health posts staffed by two volunteer CHWs each (serving areas with populations of 1,000–1,500). Starting in 2007 (1386 AC), a large number of subcenters were opened, serving populations of 3,000–7,000. The BPHS also describes in considerable detail the staffing, equipment, supplies, and types of services available at each level of care.

Although the BPHS has clearly been an important contributor to the success of the health sector in Afghanistan, a number of important challenges remain. They include providing coverage, access, and utilization; enhancing M&E of the delivery of the BPHS; balancing stewardship and managerial autonomy; and deciding on how the scope of the BPHS should continue to evolve.

The rest of this chapter discusses these four challenges and explores the options available for further strengthening the content, delivery, and utilization of the BPHS. The chapter also assesses the evidence and rationale for different approaches that have been suggested.

Improving Coverage, Access, and Utilization

Although the coverage of primary health care has increased considerably since 2002 (1381 AC), particularly in rural areas, more needs to be done. Sixty percent of the rural population still lives more than an hour's travel from any health facility, and the coverage of key preventive and health promotion services remains low by international standards. There is a rapid drop-off in skilled birth attendance as travel time from the nearest health facility increases (see figure 2.3 in chapter 2).

The issue of physical access is further complicated by sociocultural impediments that prevent women from using health services. Afghanistan's culture imposes restrictions on women's mobility and their presence in public places. This partly explains why even when health facilities are close by, only a quarter of women use skilled birth attendants. In addition to these impediments, insecurity in parts of the country appears to have a significant effect both on the ability of the MOPH and its partners to deliver the BPHS and on users' ability to access services. Thus, increasing coverage and utilization is the single largest challenge in strengthening the BPHS.

Subcenters

Subcenters are small clinics close to the community that emerged in response to difficult geography. An Afghan NGO working under a performance-based partnership agreement (PPA) in Farah province opened the first subcenters in 2005 (1384 AC), in response to lower than expected utilization of services. The NGO, Coordination of Humanitarian Assistance (CHA), believed that Afghanistan's dispersed population and difficult terrain made it necessary to establish small clinics that could provide most BPHS services closer to the community. Each subcenter established by CHA was staffed by a male nurse and a female nurse or midwife as well as a guard. Because they used rented facilities, the subcenters could be established rapidly at reasonably low cost. In 2007 (1386 AC), 125 subcenters were opened in provinces that were receiving World Bank financing. More than 100 subcenters are being financed by Global Alliance for Vaccines and Immunization (GAVI)–Health Systems Strengthening funds in other provinces.

Subcenters appear to have been successful in increasing access to BPHS services. The subcenters established in PPA and Ministry of Public Health–Strengthening Mechanism (MOPH–SM) provinces appear to have contributed to an increase in the volume of services provided, particularly in remote areas. The average subcenter provides as much as two-thirds of the outpatient visits, half the deliveries and new antenatal care services, and more than 40 percent of the family planning services provided by basic health centers. Evidence from three contiguous provinces in northern Afghanistan—Faryab, Ghor, and Sari Pul—indicates that subcenters appear to be having a net positive effect on service delivery such as outpatient visits (figure 6.1) and growth monitoring (figure 6.2). In Sari Pul, 17 subcenters were opened in the second quarter of 2007 (1386 AC); no subcenters

Figure 6.1   Trends in Annual Outpatient Visits per Capita in Three Northern Provinces, 2006/07–2007/08 (1385–86 AC)

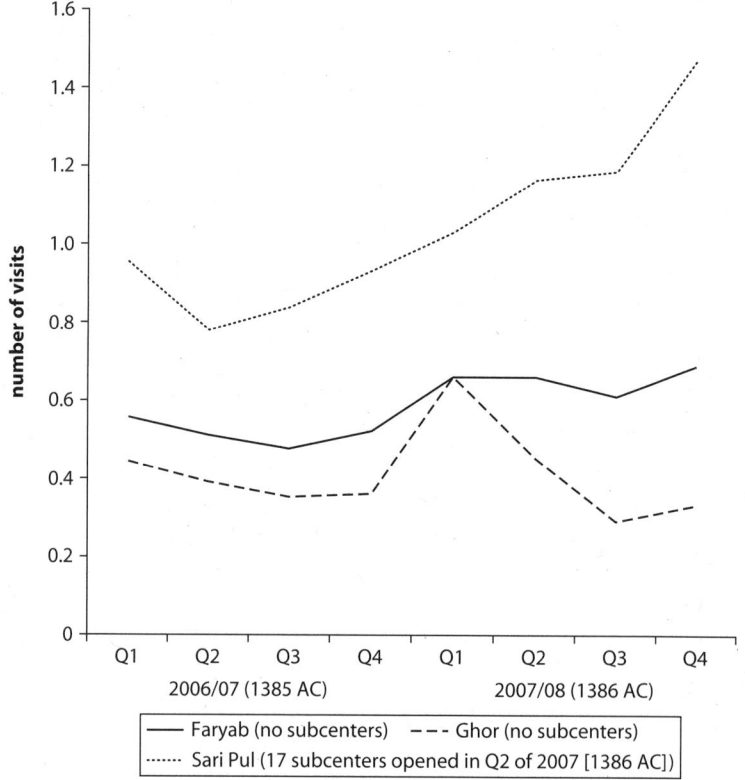

Source: Health Management Information System data (Ministry of Public Health).

Figure 6.2   Trends in Growth Monitoring Coverage in Three Northern Provinces, 2006/07–2007/08 (1385–86 AC)

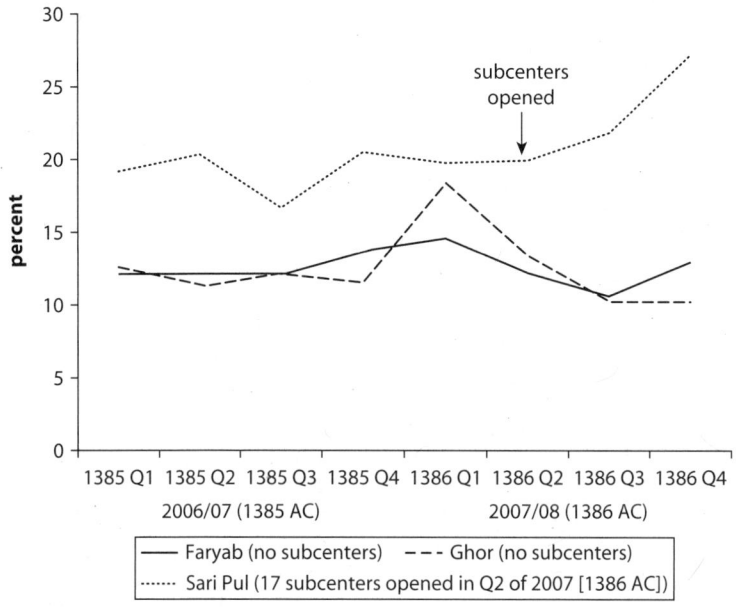

Source: Health Management Information System data (Ministry of Public Health).

were established in Faryab or Ghor. Figures 6.1 and 6.2 suggest that the increases in Sari Pul were greater than both the secular trend and the changes observed in the other two provinces.

The costs of subcenters appear reasonable relative to their benefits. The cost of operating a subcenter has been estimated at $18,000– $22,000 a year, which is considerably less than the costs of basic health centers and community health centers. On a cost-per-patient basis, subcenters are considerably more efficient than larger facilities. In addition, subcenters are important in improving equity and reaching the most remote communities, where under-five mortality rates and maternal mortality ratios are often highest. Subcenters also appear politically advantageous to the MOPH, as they provide evidence of its commitment to expand service delivery and allow the government to highlight to the population new functional facilities that did not previously exist.

Other than the cost, the main challenge in establishing additional subcenters is ensuring sufficient staff, particularly trained female staff. The most effective solution will likely be training additional community midwives or developing a new cadre of female community nurses, as suggested earlier in this volume. Concern has been expressed that subcenters could hinder the effectiveness of CHWs. Discussions with implementing NGOs, however, find no evidence that subcenters interfere with their activities. On the contrary, having health facilities closer to the communities served by CHWs appears to strengthen the linkages between CHWs and the health care system.

Initiatives for Improving Service Delivery in Insecure Areas

The most serious challenge facing the BPHS is how to deliver services in the context of worsening insecurity. There are reports that the Taliban have targeted health workers and health facilities and then told villagers that the government cannot provide them with any services. For example, in Helmand province, 12 out of 440 health workers (2.7 percent) were killed between 2006 and mid-2008 (1385–87 AC). There were 42 functioning facilities in Helmand in 2004 (1383 AC); by 2006 (1385 AC) the number had dropped to 26, a 38 percent reduction (this situation remains fluid).

The results of this insecurity are evident in health service utilization patterns. The same Afghan NGO (Ibn Sina) working in Helmand also had a PPA in Sari Pul province in northern Afghanistan, where security has been consistently better. Utilization of health services has grown much more quickly in Sari Pul (figure 6.3). Both provinces started at roughly similar levels of health facility utilization. Comparison of the two provinces is complicated, however, by the fact that Helmand is socially more conservative than Sari Pul. Data from other insecure provinces, including Kandahar, Uruzgan, and Zabul, also indicate much slower progress in increasing BPHS utilization than in the country as a whole.

NGOs are initiating creative responses to increase BPHS utilization in insecure areas. As a result of insecurity, Ibn Sina in Helmand was unable to spend much of the funds it had been given under its PPA. Working with the MOPH and local communities, it instituted a series of innovations in an attempt to improve utilization and coverage:

- A conditional cash transfer scheme, which provided families with cash when their children came for well-child visits and mothers delivered at a health facility
- A performance-based incentive scheme for CHWs that linked payments to the number of children fully immunized, the number of mothers who delivered at health facilities, and the number of tuberculosis cases detected

Figure 6.3   Trend in Annual Outpatient Visits per Capita in Secure (Sari Pul) and Insecure (Helmand) Provinces, 2004–06 (1383–85 AC)

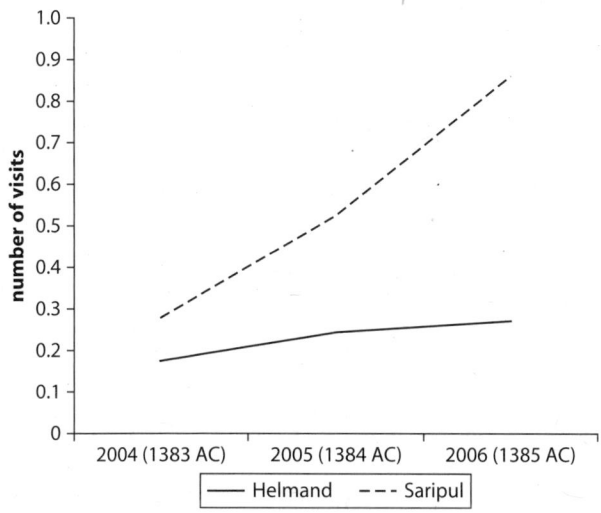

Source: Health Management Information System data (Ministry of Public Health).

- A security allowance for skilled health workers on top of the national salary policy, to keep insecure facilities well staffed
- The establishment of 10 subcenters
- Monitoring by the provincial health office and members of the community, as well as self-assessment by Ibn Sina.

Early evidence suggests that such innovations, particularly conditional cash payments, are effective in insecure areas. Shortly after the introduction of the innovations described above, a large increase in the uptake of services was reported in the Health Management Information System (HMIS) (figure 6.4). In the absence of an independent verification system, overreporting is a possibility, but efforts were made to minimize overreporting through provincial health offices and community leaders.

The innovations used in Helmand could be implemented in other insecure areas. Although the evidence for the success of these innovations is for a short period and comes primarily from the HMIS, the improvements are sufficiently dramatic to suggest that highly insecure areas in Afghanistan could also achieve large increases in utilization. Given that these innovations are relatively low cost and help NGOs use funds they might not otherwise be able to spend, implementation of this package of innovations should be replicated in other areas.

Figure 6.4   Changes in Selected Indicators in Helmand Province after Introduction of New Approaches, 2007/08–2008/09 (1386–87 AC)

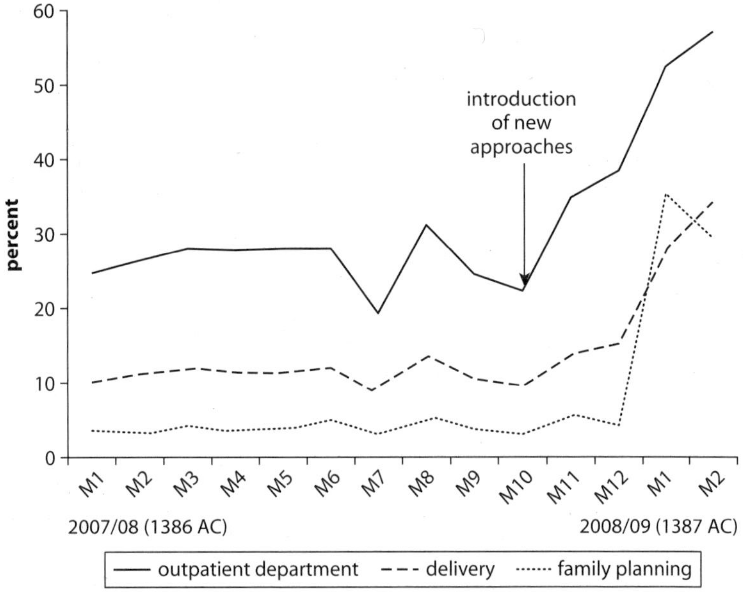

Source: Health Management Information System data (Ministry of Public Health).

Community Health Workers

The MOPH and implementing partners have trained and deployed a large number of CHWs. CHWs have been seen as a key part of the BPHS, and there are now more than 18,000 of them countrywide. Operations research carried out by Johns Hopkins University in collaboration with the MOPH (MOPH, JHU, and IIHMR 2007a) indicates that 37 percent of CHWs are women and more than 60 percent have more than six years of schooling. Sixty-four percent of BPHS facilities have active CHWs in their catchment areas, and 57 percent of the facilities have community health supervisors.

Support for CHWs has been good. The operations research—which was based on health facility assessments, interviews of CHWs, focus group discussions with members of the community, and the 2006 (1385 AC) Afghanistan Household Survey—found that the health system has been supporting CHWs well. More than 90 percent of CHWs reported receiving three or more supervisory visits in the previous six months, and more than two-thirds reported having supplies of oral rehydration salts, cotrimoxazole, and paracetamol. The training of CHWs also appears to be effective, as most of the CHWs surveyed had reasonable knowledge of basic preventive health measures.

There is some debate over what impact CHWs are actually having in their communities. The 2006 (1385AC) household survey found that only 25 percent of households were aware of a CHW in their community. In 44 percent of the clusters surveyed, no households were aware of CHWs. In addition, CHWs appear to be providing little in the way of curative care. Among family members who were ill in the previous 30 days and sought care, only 3 percent received it from a CHW. Other surveys show, however, that CHWs have indeed had some impact on maternal and child health services. Further analysis of the household data is needed to determine whether the presence of CHWs improves service delivery (such as the contraceptive prevalence rate).

Improving CHW impact may require more clearly focused job responsibilities. Although CHWs are appreciated by *shura-e-sehie* (community health committee) members, it is widely felt that the job description of CHWs is too broad. It may be worth providing strategic direction to the CHWs and getting them to focus on referring clients to health facilities for maternal and child services and changing a few key behaviors, such as increasing handwashing, appropriately using weaning foods, and increasing birth spacing. These behaviors could be affected by CHWs and would be expected to have an impact on maternal and child health outcomes.

Compensating CHWs may be necessary to improve their performance and impact. All stakeholders involved in BPHS delivery recognize the need for providing some form of payment to CHWs. Global experience with CHWs suggests that relying on volunteers leads to higher dropout rates and reduces impact (MOPH, JHU, and IIHMR 2007a). But paying even modest amounts to CHWs can be costly because of their sheer numbers. For example, providing $20 (Af. 1,000) a month would cost about $6 million a year over what is currently spent on CHWs. It is not just the number of payments and their cost that need to be considered. Linking CHW payments to actual performance (such as knowledge of handwashing in the community, as judged by the community health supervisor) might be important for increasing CHWs' impact.

Rigorous evaluation of CHW payment schemes is necessary. Given the cost of CHWs, it is important to understand how to obtain the greatest impact from the effort. The MOPH is working on a randomized study of the payment of CHW incentives that may be linked to performance. The results of this study should be used, in conjunction with an analysis of costs, to make a decision about how the CHW program should be run in the future.

Other Potentially Important Innovations

Innovations aimed at increasing the utilization of the BPHS should be field tested and evaluated. The MOPH is currently pilot testing a set of potentially effective innovations to improve the coverage and utilization of BPHS services. These innovations should be carefully evaluated to determine whether they are effective in the Afghan context at a cost that can be sustained. Successful innovations should then be scaled up. The most promising interventions include the following:

- *Mobile clinics.* The MOPH has developed an approach of using teams of mobile health workers that visit remote villages on a regular basis to deliver the BPHS. Generally, the mobile clinics have used existing vehicles, such as ambulances, to visit villages with limited access to services. There is concern among some stakeholders about the cost of such mobile clinics. Systematic evaluation of their effectiveness is necessary.

- *Demand-side incentives.* Providing cash or other incentives to patients who come to health facilities for priority services could be very important for increasing utilization of key BPHS services. Whether utilization is constrained by social values, distance, or insecurity, such demand-side payments have worked reasonably well in other countries. Experience in Afghanistan has also been very encouraging, including in Helmand province, where such payments appear to have worked well even in insecure areas. The MOPH, using GAVI funds, is in the process of rigorously testing demand-side incentives.

- *Results-based financing for health workers.* There has been some successful experience, particularly in Cambodia and Rwanda, in providing incentive payments to health workers based on the number of services they actually provide (Vujicic 2008). For example, providing payments to health workers in individual health centers for the number of deliveries attended in the facility has led to an increase in institutional deliveries. The MOPH is working with the World Bank on the design of a randomized trial of a results-based financing scheme.

Enhancing Monitoring and Evaluation of the BPHS

M&E is key to the success of the BPHS. The MOPH and its development partners have invested much time, effort, and resources in regular and independent M&E of BPHS performance through household surveys, health facility surveys, monitoring checklists, field supervision, and a strengthened HMIS, which relies on routinely recorded and reported data. This investment in M&E has allowed the MOPH and its development partners to track progress, identify problems, and ensure that implementing partners are performing well. The various sources of data have helped the MOPH monitor the availability of inputs, the quality of care provided in the field, improvements in coverage and utilization, and the impact on health outcomes. Although carrying out regular, independent, and rigorous M&E of health sector performance is relatively expensive (it accounted for about 6 percent of total expenditures in the World Bank–financed health project), it allows an evidence-based and rational approach to policy formulation to be adopted.

A standard set of BPHS indicators is needed. Although the MOPH and its development partners have agreed generally on how to judge progress of the BPHS, it would be helpful if all implementing partners used a consistent set of indicators. Afghanistan's national development strategy, health strategy, and M&E strategy use somewhat different indicators; it would be helpful for the revised BPHS to include a limited and standard set of indicators.

No single source of information is sufficient. The MOPH uses multiple sources of information effectively to "triangulate" the assessment of overall health sector performance. The various sources of data have different benefits and disadvantages, so it makes sense to use them in conjunction with one another.

- *HMIS*. The advantage of the HMIS is that it provides near real-time information and allows managers to easily track their own performance at a disaggregated level. The disadvantages of using the HMIS to monitor system performance include the following: it is very expensive if the staff time required to fill in the forms is factored in; it does not provide data on important aspects of services, such as equity, community satisfaction, health expenditure, and use of other services, particularly from the private sector; and managers or NGOs may not be concerned with data quality or overstate their performance. For example, there were significant differences between the results of the 2006 (1385 AC) Afghanistan Household Survey and the HMIS on immunization coverage and antenatal care coverage, with the HMIS showing substantially better performance.

- *Household surveys*. Household surveys, including lot quality assurance sampling, have several advantages: they are generally more accurate than other surveys; they are not dependent on information collected by local managers or NGOs; and they provide community data on coverage, equity, health care expenditures, use of the private sector, and satisfaction. The main disadvantage of household surveys is that they are relatively expensive to carry out.

- *Health facility surveys*. The MOPH has relied heavily on the results of health facility surveys, particularly the Balanced Score Card, to assess various aspects of quality of care, such as the knowledge and skills of providers; the satisfaction of patients; and the availability of inputs, including pharmaceuticals, supplies, equipment, and staff. The benefits of the health facility surveys include the following: they can assess quality of care from a technical perspective rather than based on perceptions of quality; they provide an independent assessment of what is happening in the facilities operated by NGOs and MOPH–SM; and they can be conducted frequently (annually) at reasonable cost. The disadvantage of health facility surveys is that they can motivate managers on the ground to focus too much on inputs and processes rather than coverage, utilization of services, and outcomes.

- *Supervisory checklists*. The national monitoring checklist, developed by the MOPH, is a short health facility survey that can be used to quickly and regularly track quality of care (broadly defined) in specific health facilities. The MOPH has also designed a simple checklist that members of the community can use to assess services.

- *Demographic surveillance*. The MOPH has begun developing a system of demographic surveillance that would provide annual estimates of infant mortality, under-five mortality, fertility rates, and, possibly, cause of death. Such a system would provide essential information in a more timely manner than can be obtained from household surveys (estimates of the under-five mortality rate from surveys typically lag by 2.5–3 years). The possible disadvantages of demographic surveillance are its expense (it may cost more initially to set up, although recurrent costs may be lower) and its technical and logistical complexity, especially in insecure areas.

- *Disease surveillance*. The MOPH has successfully implemented a disease early warning system (DEWS), which provides data on the incidence of specific communicable diseases and the occurrence of epidemics.

Adequate resources should be allocated to M&E, including HMIS. Given the rapidly changing (and mostly improving) nature of the health sector in Afghanistan, it will be important to ensure that the MOPH and its partners obtain reliable information frequently. The common practice is that health systems should spend about 5 percent of their total expenditure on M&E. Thus, in the case of the BPHS, it would make sense to spend about $5 million a year. This level of financing would allow collection of information using all the methods described above. Priority should be given to annual health facility assessments, biannual household surveys representative at the provincial level combined with lot quality assessment surveys in alternate years, and demographic surveillance. This approach would ensure that the MOPH and its partners continue to have the information needed for evidence-based decision making.

Data should be made publicly available. For reasons of transparency and to allow more in-depth analysis of the data collected, both reports and original data sets should be made available to the public. The MOPH should establish a policy of disseminating information within a fixed period of time (perhaps 6–12 months) after data collection is completed and asking researchers to provide copies of any analysis that uses the data. Data and reports could be made available on the MOPH Web site.

Balancing Stewardship and Managerial Autonomy

The BPHS has been central to MOPH stewardship. Before introduction of the BPHS, NGOs did not have a consistent program and often focused on very different priorities (some emphasized infectious disease control, others reproductive health, and still others noncommunicable disease control). The various NGOs also established different types of facilities and used different types of staff. The BPHS has helped ensure that there is a consistent, national set of priorities and common overall approach. In particular, it has helped ensure a focus on key health interventions (the "what" of health services).

Providing managers with significant autonomy has had clear advantages. Through the BPHS, the MOPH has provided a clear strategy to the sector and its implementing partners. However, the MOPH has generally given managers at the provincial level substantial independence in how to manage and organize service delivery (the "how" of health service delivery). Giving managers on the ground considerable autonomy has had many advantages, including the following:

- Management decisions are made by the people who are closest to the ground reality and who can make the most informed decisions about how to tackle problems that arise (for example, how to ensure sufficient female staff).
- It is easier for the MOPH to hold managers accountable for results, because they cannot claim that the actions, or inaction, of others interfered with their performance (for example, if a manager is responsible for procurement of pharmaceuticals and supplies or recruitment of staff, he cannot blame anyone else if there is a shortage).
- Management autonomy allows and actually encourages innovations that can improve performance (for example, the establishment of subcenters arose because of managerial autonomy).
- Managers can avoid rigid government rules and regulations that often hinder flexible solutions to even mundane issues (for example, in MOPH–SM provinces managers cannot easily buy tea and biscuits for members of the *shura-e-sehie*).
- Managers are able to avoid excessive political interference, which might otherwise result in irrational and inefficient management decisions.

Decentralizing management functions improves results. There are a few areas in which there have been variations in the approaches to specific management functions. For example, drug procurement has been decentralized to NGOs in PPA provinces but centralized in performance-based partnership grant (PPG) and MOPH–SM provinces. Decentralized procurement has improved the availability of pharmaceuticals in health facilities, as indicated by the drug availability index (table 6.1). Independent assessment has not found any issues of poor drug quality (MOPH, JHU, and IIHMR 2007b).

Priorities should be set centrally, but management functions should be decentralized. Programmatic priorities should be determined by the MOPH centrally, based on careful analysis of the evidence. However, how service delivery is organized and managed should be left to the managers who will be held responsible for the results. For example, specifying that immunization is a priority and that coverage should increase is important and sensible. Indicating how immunization services should be delivered is not: whether NGO contractors want to go house to house, stand on street corners, or set up mobile clinics in schools should be left up to them.

Table 6.1   Drug Availability Index, by Type of Procurement, 2004 (1383 AC) and 2007 (1386 AC)

Type of procurement	2004 (1383 AC)	2007 (1386 AC)	Change 2004–07 (1383–86 AC) (percent)
Decentralized NGO procurement (PPA)	58.0	93.9	36.0
Centralized procurement (MOPH–SM)	58.0	88.8	30.8
Centralized procurement (PPG)	67.0	81.4	14.4

Source: Balanced Score Card (Ministry of Public Health 2008a).
Note: Index ranges from 0 to 100. MOPH-SM = Ministry of Public Health-Strengthening Mechanism; NGO = non-governmental organization; PPA = performance-based partnership agreement; PPG = performance-based partnership grant.

What matters is that coverage increases, not how it is achieved. The two exceptions to this principle should be cases in which there is strong scientific evidence for a particular approach to how services are delivered and cases in which it is important to ensure that implementing partners comply with national technical standards regarding quality of care. For example, based on evidence from an experiment, the MOPH decided to prohibit user fees (implementation has been far from ideal); NGOs must follow and not alter the national schedule for child immunization (for example, they should immunize children with measles vaccine at 9 months and not change it to 6 months or 15 months).

The default position should be leaving management decisions to managers on the ground. One of the problems with centralized decision making has been that such decisions tend to take a long time. For example, the central MOPH took more than 10 months to decide whether the post of community health supervisor should be added to the staffing of basic health centers. This is the type of decision that would be best left up to NGO managers at the provincial level. Taking into account the advantages of decentralized management, the default position should be that when it comes to how health services are delivered and managed, decisions should be left up to NGO or MOPH–SM managers. The MOPH should intervene as little as possible in management and organization decisions—and then only when there is compelling scientific evidence supporting a certain approach. Personnel and logistics management should usually be decentralized.

Vertical programs have an important role to play. Vertical programs, such as the Expanded Program on Immunization (EPI) or the tuberculosis and malaria programs, concentrate on supporting specific activities by setting technical standards and guidelines, conducting training, carrying out supervision, and defining reporting requirements. They also provide supplies (such as vaccines, tuberculosis drug blister packs, and insecticide-treated nets) that are otherwise not readily available.

In most developing countries, there is a tension between vertical programs and the managers responsible for delivering health services in the field. This tension can be creative, but it can also impede delivery of the BPHS unless clear principles are laid out. There are already examples of situations in which vertical program staff at the provincial level, in their desire to push the program, have interfered with and duplicated the efforts of managers charged with implementing the BPHS. In other countries, serious conflicts have arisen (for example, HIV/AIDS programs have taken over some staff in health facilities and paid them more than other staff). Avoiding these issues will help ensure overall MOPH stewardship.

Vertical programs should generally not limit managerial autonomy if the MOPH ensures that there are no vertical program staff below the level of province, no incentives are paid by vertical programs (or their donors) to staff below the provincial level to work on a particular program (for example, the tuberculosis program should not give incentives or salary supplements to health workers for providing tuberculosis treatment); and the number of vertical program staff in the provincial health office is kept to a modest level (a maximum of two to three per program).

The MOPH should also ensure that vertical programs and their staff refrain from telling field managers how to organize or manage health services. Managers are responsible for service delivery and have more insight into how things are working on the ground. (EPI staff, for example, should focus on the "what" of service delivery by ensuring that high coverage is being achieved, the vaccination schedule is being followed, and the cold chain is being properly maintained. They should not tell managers how to organize EPI services.) Finally, the MOPH should ensure that new reporting requirements by vertical programs are approved by the M&E department.

Prioritizing Interventions for Inclusion in the BPHS

Regularly updating the BPHS makes sense. The MOPH is about to complete the process of revising the BPHS, with a focus on what new interventions, if any, should be added. Revising the BPHS every five years or so is sensible, so that new technologies, new data, and new experience can be reflected in its content.

Given resource constraints, interventions should be added carefully. Including new interventions in the BPHS will cost money and will therefore compete for the same limited resources as other mechanisms for increasing its impact, such as establishing additional subcenters, increasing support to CHWs, providing demand-side payments, and carrying out M&E. Because financial resource constraints are real and serious, adding new interventions to the BPHS should be done carefully. Caution should also be used in expanding BPHS interventions in order not to diminish the value of having clearly enunciated priorities and tarnishing the "brand recognition" the BPHS has earned. Adding too many services to the BPHS may also result in a loss of focus on interventions that are currently being implemented but still require strengthening (for example, skilled birth attendance in 2006 [1385 AC] stood at only 19 percent, and the contraceptive prevalence rate was only 15 percent).

Adding interventions to the BPHS should be based on specific criteria. A limited set of criteria, such as the following, should be applied to any proposed addition:

- The efficacy of the intervention should be clear, and the quality of the scientific evidence supporting it should be rigorous.
- The burden of disease prevented or cured by the intervention should be large.
- The intervention should be easy to implement in Afghanistan, as judged by pilot implementation under field conditions.
- The intervention should be low cost and cost-effective compared with other interventions.
- Consistent with the overall objectives of the government and the MOPH as expressed in the Afghanistan national development strategy and the health and nutrition policy, the intervention should provide disproportionate benefit to children, women, and the poor.
- The intervention should be deliverable through the primary health care system.

The government has clearly prioritized maternal and child health in the national development strategy and identified the reduction of under-five mortality rates and maternal mortality ratios as key indicators of success. To be consistent with its policies, new additions to the BPHS should focus on improving maternal and child health. They should address the primary causes of under-five and maternal mortality.

Although different observers may have different perceptions, the above criteria suggest a few other interventions that should be considered for inclusion in the BPHS:

• *Rotavirus and streptococcal vaccines.* These vaccines address the major causes of death in children in Afghanistan: diarrhea and acute respiratory infections. Although these vaccines are expensive, they may be particularly important in insecure areas, where children may not be able to benefit from early treatment of these diseases.

• *Behavior change focused on a few key behaviors.* To be effective, behavior change communication needs to focus on changing only a few specific behaviors that will have a strong impact on maternal and child health. The messages related to the selected behaviors need to be carefully thought through and tested, then repeated frequently using various media (including interpersonal communication). The data measuring which behavior changes will have the most impact identify three interventions as key: increasing handwashing by mothers and young children, which would be expected to have a large impact on the incidence of diarrhea and acute respiratory infections; encouraging appropriate weaning, starting at 4–6 months, with increased caloric intake; and promoting birth spacing (children born with a birth interval of less than 24 months run more than twice the risk of dying in childhood borne by children born after longer intervals).

• *Postpartum visits.* Neonatal mortality in Afghanistan, which likely accounts for only about 20 percent of under-five mortality, could be reduced by some simple and effective interventions. Visits by skilled health workers 24–48 hours after delivery, with the possibility of initiating treatment for sepsis or pneumonia, may be particularly effective.

A broadly consultative and scientific process should be used in revising the BPHS. In order to have widespread buy-in, the revision should be based on a broad consultative process that involves all stakeholders concerned with financing health sector investments, including the Ministry of Finance and development partners. Although advocates for specific interventions should be heard, they should not have the dominant voice in making decisions. Contentious interventions should be carefully evaluated by pilot tests before being incorporated into the BPHS.

Concluding Remarks: Findings and Recommendations

The BPHS has been central to the success of the health sector in Afghanistan, because it has provided a strategic focus on high-impact interventions, ensured that resources are allocated equitably, and established a basic structure for service delivery in the health sector. This success notwithstanding, the BPHS faces important challenges, including the need to improve coverage and utilization, further strengthen M&E, balance the stewardship function of the MOPH with autonomy for managers, and determine which, if any, interventions to add.

Improving Coverage, Access, and Utilization

Given that 60 percent of Afghans live more than one hour's travel from a health facility, improving access is a high priority. Subcenters that provide the BPHS to 3,000–7,000 people have been successful in increasing coverage of services; their number should be expanded by at least a few hundred. Ibn Sina has implemented a series of innovations in Helmand province, including a conditional cash payment scheme that appears to have had a dramatic impact on utilization of services in a very insecure environment. These measures have been shown to be successful and should be replicated in other insecure areas.

Many CHWs have been deployed, but only 25 percent of households are aware of their presence in their community, raising questions about their impact. Increasing their impact may require that CHWs focus on a few strategic priorities and be paid a performance-linked stipend. These approaches need to be rigorously field tested. Other innovations—including mobile clinics, demand-side payments, and results-based financing for health workers—should also be field tested and evaluated.

Enhancing Monitoring and Evaluation

Given the dynamic nature of the health sector in Afghanistan and the challenges it faces, further strengthening M&E will be key if policymaking is to be informed by evidence. No single source of information is sufficient. If the MOPH and its partners allocate about 5 percent of BPHS expenditures to M&E, the sector could afford to obtain data through biannual household surveys at the provincial level (with lot quality assessment surveys in alternate years), annual health facility assessments, and demographic surveillance. Data from these sources should also be made public, including through the MOPH's Web site.

Balancing Stewardship and Managerial Autonomy

The BPHS has been a central part of MOPH stewardship over the health sector, particularly when it comes to setting priorities. By providing MOPH–SM and NGO managers with considerable autonomy, the MOPH has ensured that difficult management issues, such as logistics and staffing, have been successfully addressed. Based on the experience thus far, it makes sense that decisions about how health services are delivered and managed be left up to managers on the ground. In order to keep an appropriate balance between vertical programs and field managers, there should be no vertical program staff below the provincial level, no incentives should be paid by vertical programs, and all reporting requirements should be approved by the M&E department.

Contracting of BPHS provision to MOPH–SM and NGOs needs to continue. It has proven enormously successful in expanding service coverage. Results from comparative analyses show that both PPA and PPG contracting perform much better at expanding service and improving quality of care than regular MOPH provision (Belay 2009). The MOPH should expand this contracting model.

Prioritizing Interventions to Add to the BPHS

There will always be the temptation to add to the BPHS. However, it is critical that the BPHS remain focused on addressing a limited number of health interventions that address key health problems with the highest disease burden. Any revision needs to be done carefully, given resource constraints, and should be based on specific criteria, including the strength of the evidence, the ease of implementation, and the cost. Based on these criteria, salt iodination; administration of rotavirus and streptococcal vaccines; and behavior change communication focused on handwashing, weaning practices, and birth spacing could be considered.

CHAPTER 7

Institutional Capacity of the Ministry of Public Health

The Ministry of Public Health (MOPH) has emerged as a highly capable body that has overseen remarkable progress in the health system. This progress has been achieved largely through a focus on stewardship functions and limited involvement in the direct provision of health services. The strong stewardship role that the MOPH has played since 2004 (1383 AC) has contributed to important gains in health for the Afghan population.

Despite this impressive performance over the past several years, many challenges continue to threaten the performance of the health sector. The health and nutrition sector strategy highlights the following as the main challenges Afghanistan faces in continuing to improve its population's health:

- Lack of qualified staff, especially female staff, at all levels of the health system
- Lack of secure and predictable funding of the health system, which is heavily reliant on donors
- Inadequate coordination with NGOs providing services
- Insufficient investments at the provincial level
- Inadequate investment in health management information systems (HMIS) and monitoring and evaluation (M&E) capacity.

All of these issues are directly related to strengthening the stewardship functions of the MOPH.

This chapter identifies the functions of the MOPH, addresses specific questions related to each function (based on data from the institutional survey; see box 7.1), and identifies gaps in order to better prepare the ministry to carry out its stewardship functions. The institutional analysis covers the major stewardship responsibilities, including setting the strategic direction of the health sector, coordinating donors, mobilizing resources, accrediting and regulating the private sector, promoting behavior changes of public health importance, and conducting M&E. The chapter assesses the skills that the MOPH will require to carry out these functions effectively and the organizational and institutional arrangements, including subnational structures, needed to help facilitate these functions. Functions related to regulation of the private sector and human resources for health are addressed in chapters 4 and 5 and are not covered here.

The rest of the chapter presents the results of the institutional assessment of the MOPH. The performance of the MOPH is assessed under each of the identified functions. Key findings and recommendations are provided for each function.

Setting Strategies and Objectives

The process through which MOPH policies, strategies, rules, and regulations are developed is clear to MOPH officials. Generally, policies, strategies, and guidelines are developed by task forces and working groups formed by the MOPH for this purpose. After scrutiny by the concerned departments, the documents are presented to the Consultative Group on Health and Nutrition (CGHN) for comments and approval by stakeholders in the health sector.[1] The CGHN then forwards the approved document to the Technical Advisory Group (TAG), a group of internal and external advisors that submits recommendations to the ministry's Executive Board for endorsement or further review and comments. Finally, the documents are presented to the MOPH Executive Board—the highest decision-making body in the MOPH, chaired by His Excellency the Minister of Public Health—for final approval.

The MOPH has developed a large number of policies, strategies, and technical guidelines. The General Directorate for Policy and Planning

Box 7.1

Issues Addressed under Each Function of the Ministry of Public Health

- *Setting strategies and objectives.* Are the different strategy documents (the Afghanistan national development strategy, the health and nutrition policy, and so forth) consistent? Do they include the same indicators of success? Are they easy to understand? Do MOPH staff (and other stakeholders) know what the strategies are? Do they know what the indicators of success are? Is there agreement between the central MOPH and provincial health offices (PHOs)?
- *Budget preparation and resource mobilization.* Is there an effective strategy for mobilizing resources? Does the MOPH proactively mobilize resources? Does the budgeting process constrain efforts to mobilize resources?
- *Monitoring, evaluation, and use of data.* Do managers know how their province is doing on key indicators? Do they take actions based on results? Does the information collected meet managers' needs?
- *Accountability and responsiveness.* How does the MOPH (and its PHOs) communicate its policies and operations to the public? Are financial and service utilization data made available to the public? What are the constraints on making information available?
- *Technical guidelines and supervision.* Are technical guidelines sensible and based on international best practice? Have they been properly vetted by technical peers? Do they take into account cost implications? Are they widely available? Do managers focus on what is getting done rather than how it is getting done? Do they know and understand the technical guidelines? Are they using the national supervisory checklist?
- *Coordination of development partners.* Are coordination meetings focused on results? Are decisions made to improve services? Are decisions properly followed up?
- *Information, education, and communication/behavior change communication (IEC/BCC).* Is there a clear IEC/BCC objective, including what behaviors need to be changed?
- *Emergency response.* Does the MOPH have staff trained in emergency response? Does it have plans for dealing with emergencies? Has it practiced its emergency response?

(GDPP), which coordinates the development of policies and strategies, has carried out a mapping of the current documents to identify gaps, accelerate the development and approval of (draft) documents, and plan for the renewal of outdated policies and strategies.

There are differences between basic package of health services (BPHS) and essential package of hospital services (EPHS) documents in terms of mission statements and goals. Comparison of the principal MOPH policy documents—namely, the "National Health Policy 2005–2009 (1384–87 AC)" and the Health and Nutrition Sector Strategy of the "Afghanistan National Development Strategy 1387–1391 (2007/08–2012/13)"—reveals that the BPHS and the EPHS form the backbone of both documents (Ministry of Public Health 2005, 2008c). Neither document contains a list of national indicators or targets for the various components of the health system. Both present the desired outcomes, although the outcomes vary slightly. The desired outcomes listed in the "National Health Policy 2005–2009 (1384–87 AC)" are reduction in maternal, under-five, and infant mortality and reduction of malnutrition among children under five years of age. The desired outcomes listed in the health and nutrition sector strategy are increased access to health services; reduction in maternal, under-five, and infant mortality; and increases in measles and diphtheria, pertussis, and tetanus (DPT3) coverage. The list of national priority health indicators and the MOPH factsheet are given in another document, the "Strategic Plan for Monitoring and Evaluation 1386–1390" (2007–11) (Ministry of Public Health 2007). This document has not been disseminated to the staff of the MOPH, provincial health offices (PHOs), NGOs, or other partners.

Dissemination within the MOPH

The MOPH has been extremely successful in disseminating its key documents to NGOs and donors but not in disseminating them to its own departments and provincial offices. The Health Economics and Finance Directorate (the former Grants and Contracts Management Unit) and the MOPH Resource Center play a critical role in dissemination. However, all respondents reported that there was no effective mechanism for distributing and explaining new MOPH policies, strategies, and guidelines to MOPH departments or PHOs. Only respondents from the provinces covered by the Tech-Serve project declared that they received documents in a regular and timely fashion (from Tech-Serve).[2] Resource centers similar to the one inside the ministry have been established in those provinces.

The forums used for dissemination are not effective in reaching the central and provincial MOPH staff. Knowledge about MOPH policies and strategies is weak among lower-ranking staff at the central MOPH and among PHO staff of remote provinces. Knowledge of newly developed documents seems to be more uncertain among provincial officials, particularly officials who work in remote provinces and do not visit the MOPH frequently.

PHO staff had an opportunity to learn about the newly developed documents during the provincial quarterly workshops. The workshops have not been held for almost a year, however, and they were attended only by senior provincial health officials, leaving out the rest of the PHO staff. In the absence of these quarterly workshops, the MOPH has no mechanism for sharing documents with the provinces. In the past, the General Directorate of Provincial Public Health (GDPPH) (downgraded to the Provincial Health Liaison Office in the new organogram) appears to have been responsible for distributing new policies, strategies, and guidelines to the PHOs. However, its own staff are sometimes unaware of new developments inside the ministry.

The six sources of information on new policies and strategies cited by respondents are meetings of the National Technical Coordination Committee (NTCC), an information-sharing coordination body, attended by senior staff of the MOPH, donors, UN agencies, and NGOs; internal meetings of the MOPH general directorates; quarterly provincial health workshops; CGHN meetings; quarterly sector CGHN meetings on the Afghanistan national development strategy; and Executive Board meetings of the MOPH. Most of these forums are either mechanisms for coordinating with partners or decision-making bodies within the ministry.

Despite the use of these forums, in the absence of a formal distribution mechanism, MOPH staff usually learn about new policies through their own searches and contacts. Table 7.1 highlights the weaknesses of each source of information noted by survey respondents.

Involvement in the Policy Formulation Process

The policy formulation process seems participatory at the central level. Most MOPH officials indicated that they are involved in developing policies and strategies, although the level of their involvement varies. Most officials have taken part only in the development of policies and strategies related to their own work through departmental task forces and working groups. Senior officials seem to be participating in almost all policy developments of the ministry, through the TAG, the CGHN, and the Executive Board.

Table 7.1 Shortcomings of Sources of Information about New Policies of the Ministry of Public Health

Source of information	Shortcoming
NTCC meetings	Irregular attendance PHOs not represented
Internal meetings of the MOPH general directorates	Not held regularly
Quarterly provincial health workshops	Not held for almost a year
	Open only to senior provincial health officials
CGHN meetings (small)	General directorates usually absent
CGHN meetings (large)	Not held for a long time
Quarterly sector CGHN meetings on the Afghanistan national development strategy	Not held recently

Source: Author.
Note: CGHN = Consultative Group on Health and Nutrition; MOPH = Ministry of Public Health; NTCC = National Technical Coordination Committee; PHO = provincial health office.

By contrast, none of the PHOs participated directly in the development of MOPH policies and strategies. The quarterly provincial health workshops were the only place where PHOs could share their comments and raise issues for policy decisions. Some provincial health directors noted that although not involving the PHOs in policy development might have been justified because of their lack of capacity at the beginning, their capacity is now adequate, and there is no longer any reason not to involve them.

Views on MOPH Policies and Strategies

Key documents are clear and readily accessible to MOPH staff, and they are perceived as very relevant. All respondents from the central MOPH and PHOs were familiar with the key MOPH documents, and almost all of them indicated that the BPHS, the EPHS, the national health policy and strategy, and the community-based health care strategy were the most important documents developed by the MOPH. All respondents appreciated the relevance of these documents to their work and noted that they are easy to understand.

Recently developed policies are less clear and are perceived to be less relevant. Overall, the level of agreement with MOPH policies and strategies, particularly with the BPHS, the EPHS, and the national health policy and strategy, was extremely high. However, some recently developed policies and strategies (for example, those related to the control of diarrheal diseases) were heavy on background explanation but light on guidance for implementation.

A number of concerns remain about the revision of the BPHS and its sustained implementation. Some provincial officials pointed out that revision of the BPHS should address the need for more community health workers (CHWs) for remote provinces and the provision of a formal salary or incentives for CHWs. These officials also criticized the early introduction of some interventions that require more qualified human resources, which are in severe shortage even in the capitals of the provinces. Finally, some provincial officials raised concern about the sustainability of the BPHS program, which is largely dependent on foreign aid.

Budget Preparation and Resource Mobilization

Budget preparation is done by two separate departments, with little coordination. The ordinary budget is prepared by the General Directorate of Administration (GDA); the development budget is prepared by the GDPP. The Finance Department, which falls under the GDA, prepares the MOPH's ordinary budget without substantial involvement from the general directorates or the PHOs. Almost the entire GDA, including the Finance Department, has been left out of the Priority Reform Restructuring process, a national program led by the Civil Service Commission for reforming the government at all levels.[3] The GDA therefore lags behind other directorates in developing capacity and carrying out its functions effectively. Preparation of the development budget for the entire ministry is spearheaded by the GDPP, which has been active in securing funds by mobilizing donors, reducing costs, and working with the Ministry of Finance and the Afghanistan National Development Strategy Office.

Involvement in Budget Preparation

The budget preparation process is not participatory at either the central or the provincial levels. Central MOPH departments are minimally involved in the ordinary budget development process, and only a few general directors informally influence the budget process. The PHOs usually prepare annual plans and budgets, but officials described them as a waste of time, as the Finance Department of the MOPH allocates resources to the provinces based on historical expenditures, without taking into account the plans, needs, or budgets prepared by the PHOs.

Knowledge about the Available Budget

Departments are rarely informed about their budgets. Only a few central MOPH officials knew the budgets of their own programs. All of them mentioned that their departments do not have separate operational budgets, as the budget is developed for the entire ministry, without a breakdown for directorates or departments. The budgets of the PHOs are often combined with the budgets of hospitals, making it impossible for PHO officials to know exactly what financial resources they have.

Budget Execution

Budget execution is very weak, which is mainly attributed to the centralization of financial decision making within the MOPH. All MOPH staff complained about the difficulty of spending money because of their lack of financial authority and complicated MOPH and Ministry of Finance procurement and administrative procedures. Unlike NGOs, which retain financial flexibility, the MOPH maintains extremely centralized financial authority inside its own institutions. Only the minister, deputy ministers, the general director of administration, and the general director of policy and planning have financial authority. The financial authority of the two general directors is up to $2,000. The provincial health directors also have limited financial authority.

MOPH departments have to prepare requests regarding their needs for stationery, fuel, and similar items. Each request has to be approved by line officers, directors, and general directors before being presented to the highest-ranking manager with financial authority in the MOPH. Once approved by senior management, the request goes to the GDA, where the actual purchase of the requested item starts—after several signatures by directors and officers. If the price of the requested items exceeds $25, a committee must be established, which requires another authorization from senior management. As a result of these lengthy procedures, items are either not purchased or purchased only after long delays (on average, requests are met only after six months).

The level of centralization remains high even at the provincial level. The PHOs face the same limitations in spending their budgets as the MOPH. If a PHO needs an item, it has to submit a request to the provincial governorate. After approval, the governorate establishes a purchasing or bidding committee with members from various sectors, depending on the price of the item, and forwards the request to Mostofiat, the representative of the Ministry of Finance at the provincial level. The committee procures the item, stores it, and reports to the governorate. The governorate approves the purchase and sends the approval to Mostofiat. The PHO receives the item once the process is cleared by Mostofiat. For items costing more than $1,000, procurement needs to be done in Kabul and usually takes three to six months. Despite this lengthy and complicated process, PHOs surprisingly manage to spend 60–90 percent of their budgets. This is probably because salaries constitute a considerable proportion of the budget.

Available Resources

Limited resources, together with a lack of information on available resources, are a major problem. In addition to problems of execution, lack of information about the budget and lack of financial authority have severely curtailed the ability of managers in the MOPH and PHOs to set targets and plan, implement, and evaluate their activities. Some directorates—including the Afghan Public Health Institute, the Health Economics and Finance Directorate, the HMIS Unit, the Monitoring and Evaluation Department, and the Quality Assurance Department—have developmental resources at their disposal to meet their requirements. However, most MOPH departments and PHOs do not have operating budgets with which to pay for transportation, per diems, and related items.

There was widespread complaint that the per diem paid by the government is not adequate to cover costs. Some provincial officials also complained about the lack of vehicles and fuel, which left them dependent on NGOs for field visits. In addition, the budgets for the PHOs and regional hospitals are not separated, which leads to competition for available resources. There were large differences across provinces in terms of their budgets, largely because the budgets of the EPHS and regional hospitals are included in the PHO budgets. This mixed budget is probably an important factor contributing to tensions between hospital directors and PHOs.

Resource Mobilization

Some departments and provinces are directly involved in mobilizing resources, but most remain dependent on the MOPH. Although most MOPH and PHO officials said they were not actively raising developmental funds for their programs, some highlighted their active participation in fundraising activities. Some MOPH departments, including the Afghan Public Health Institute and PHOs like the one in Bamyan, attract funds and resources—for purposes ranging from purchasing stationery to constructing health facilities—through direct interaction with donors and other sources. The reasons for lack of involvement in fundraising include lack of knowledge or awareness of such opportunities (some managers were not aware that they could raise funds for their programs), lack of negotiation and proposal-writing skills, lack of strategy and guidelines, and the inability to spend the available budget.

Monitoring, Evaluation, and Use of Data

The MOPH uses several sources of information. The main sources for M&E are the Balanced Score Card, monthly HMIS reports submitted by NGOs, quarterly reports submitted by NGOs, household surveys, reports from vertical programs, and surveillance data (the 2003 multiple indicator cluster survey and the national risk and vulnerability assessment surveys, conducted by the Central Statistics Office in 2005 and 2007, and the national health household survey conducted by the Johns Hopkins Bloomberg School of Public Health in 2006). The main departments dealing with data collection and analysis in the MOPH—including the M&E Department, the Health Economics and Finance Directorate, the HMIS, and the Disease Early Warning System (DEWS) Department—are located in the GDPP and the Afghan Public Health Institute. The "Strategic Plan for Monitoring and Evaluation 1386–1390" (2007–11), which includes the national list of priority health indicators, has been prepared, but as of 2009 (1388 AC), it had not been published or formally distributed.

In general, knowledge of program indicators and use of data are common at the MOPH, although there is variation across programs. The level of awareness of program indicators and the use of information for decision making are not uniform across directorates. Officials from the vertical programs, particularly the Expanded Program on Immunization (EPI), have substantial knowledge of their indicators of success and know how their programs are performing compared with targets, although there is little information sharing with other departments of the ministry. The same is true for officials from the GDPP, where different sources of data are used, including the Balanced Score Card, the HMIS, and quarterly reports submitted by NGOs. Meetings are held with NGOs, action plans are made, and proper follow-up is done. However, many MOPH offices do not receive information from the HMIS or Balanced Score Card reports.

The use of data during management meetings for performance assessments at the central level is less frequent. In addition, the meetings at which the findings are supposed to be presented and discussed—Executive Board meetings, internal meetings of the general directorates, and quarterly provincial health workshops—are not held regularly, and when they are held, a discussion of results is usually not on the agenda. Finally, according to one official, some of the managers in the central MOPH and PHOs are so busy with meetings and the signing of too many papers that they do not have the time to look at data.

At the provincial level, data used for performance assessment are highly correlated with technical assistance for PHOs. In the provinces, the use of information and discussions about the results of Provincial Health Coordination Committee (PHCC) meetings varies from province to province.[4] The level of data use appears highest and the discussion of results most frequent in provinces in which technical assistance has been provided. In these provinces, data are used to identify weaknesses and gaps in services, action plans are made to address the problems, and plans are followed up at subsequent meetings. PHOs provide feedback, even to health facilities.

The picture is mixed for the remaining provinces. In some, there is a high level of data use for making decisions; in others, officials depend heavily on NGOs for HMIS data analysis, because qualified HMIS officers usually leave the PHOs in search of better pay. These officials also complained that they do not receive HMIS feedback from the MOPH regularly and that NGOs are sometimes not cooperative, not sharing their activity or financial reports. For some officials, understanding the Balanced Score Card is difficult, so their discussions and decisions are usually based instead on informal community feedback and direct monitoring.

In addition to technical assistance, a summary sheet on the performance of provinces would increase the use of existing data. One of the factors limiting the use of data is the lack of a standardized summary sheet, based on various sources of information (such as NGO quarterly reports, HMIS data, and the Balanced Scorecard) showing the performance of the provinces. The HMIS Unit sends compact disks (CDs) of compiled HMIS databases to all stakeholders, including the MOPH directorates, but most directorates and PHOs do not receive the CDs; when they do, they lack the capacity to analyze the data themselves.

Several concerns were raised about various data sources, especially the Balanced Score Card. Issues raised by officials from the central MOPH and PHOs include the following:

- The timing of data collection for the Balanced Score Card is known beforehand by implementing partners. This may prompt them to improve their services just before data collection.
- Because of security concerns, in some provinces data collection is done by PHO or former NGO staff.
- The Balanced Score Card is still not used widely across the MOPH or among partners, including NGOs and donors.
- Many officials at the MOPH and PHOs still have difficulty understanding the reports and presentations. According to one provincial

official, the Balanced Score Card brings excitement for a month when it is released, and then everything continues to be the same afterward. Another provincial official mentioned the Balanced Score Card findings are almost never discussed.

• There is a long gap between data collection and the release of reports, so that findings are sometimes no longer relevant. In a few instances, assessing the performance of implementing partners, based on subjective information provided by MOPH and PHO staff, is prone to various influences and motives that have put in doubt the legitimacy of the Balanced Score Card.

Accountability and Responsiveness

This section describes the ways in which the MOPH communicates its policies and operations to the public. It then identifies constraints on information sharing and assesses public opinion.

Communication of Policies and Operations to the Public

Provision of information to the public at the central level is coordinated by the Office of the Minister and the Public Relations Department of the MOPH. It occurs through press conferences and press releases, weekly meetings at the MOPH with parliamentarians, interviews with the media, and the MOPH Web site (www.MOPH.gov.af). The information shared through these channels relates to policies, strategies, achievements, and emergencies. MOPH officials also present the ministry's overall budget figures and achievements to the parliament and media on demand.

Information for the public at the provincial level is provided by the PHOs at their own initiative, with no clear guidelines. The extent of information sharing to the public and the methods used, therefore, vary considerably across provinces. The extent to which these strategies are effective and differ from province to province is not clear. At the provincial level, public health officials share information with the public through an array of channels including provincial councils, provincial coordination committees, local media, national solidarity program committees, and various types of health committees.

Constraints on Information Sharing

Although MOPH leadership is committed to providing information to the public, it has no policy or guidelines on information sharing. Other constraints include limited coordination among MOPH spokespersons;

lack of information technology (IT) capacity in terms of both human resources and infrastructure (as a result, the MOPH Web site is available only in English, severely limiting its accessibility to the general public); and lack of designated resources at the provincial level for information sharing.

Assessment of Public Opinion

The only formal mechanism by which the MOPH collects data on public opinion about its performance is the consumer satisfaction section of the annual health facility survey. The MOPH assesses the perceptions of communities about their services and the level of their satisfaction annually through the Balanced Score Card. Informally, central and provincial officials gather information through their interactions with parliamentarians, provincial councils, community committees, and the general public. The MOPH also interacts with the media regularly at the central level.

Technical Guidelines and Supervision

This section identifies weaknesses in accessibility and technical supervision. It then describes use of the national monitoring checklist.

Accessibility

There are gaps in technical guidelines, and existing guidelines remain inaccessible to provincial offices. The technical guidelines go through the same process as the policy and strategy documents in the central MOPH, without any involvement of the PHOs. To the extent that they were available and could be reviewed, it was evident that they were based on standard World Health Organization (WHO) guidelines. Areas without formal guidelines include mental health; disability; information, education, and communication; and standard treatment guidelines for hospitals.

Knowledge of relevant guidelines is limited. Although senior MOPH officials are knowledgeable about the guidelines for their programs, PHO officials, particularly officials from remote provinces, lack training on relevant guidelines except for those on the HMIS and reproductive health. Provincial officials who have not received training have limited knowledge regarding technical guidelines.

Technical Supervision

Supervision by PHO officials is not conducted regularly. The frequency of supervision and monitoring visits made by PHO officials varies considerably across provinces, depending on the availability of transportation and staff, road conditions, and security conditions. Many officials from the provinces complained about the lack of vehicles and fuel, making them dependent on the NGOs for field visits. Provinces supported by the U.S. Agency of International Development (USAID) receive the highest number of visits by consultants from the ministry, followed by MOPH–SM provinces. The general impression was that the frequency of the monitoring visits to the field had declined, because of deteriorating security, lack of transportation, low per diem reimbursements, and the heavy workload of officials at the central MOPH.

Several departments are involved in supervision work, but none focuses on technical supervision. MOPH officials regularly monitor the implementation of the BPHS across the country. However, the monitoring appears to be carried out in an uncoordinated manner and without a checklist. Various directorates and departments—including the Provincial Health Liaison Office (the former GDPPH), the Health Economics and Finance Directorate, and the M&E Department—are involved in supervision. For example, officials from the Provincial Liaison Office, whose responsibility is to support PHOs, supervise NGO–run BPHS facilities without having information about the contractual obligations of the implementing partners or the wider context in which the NGOs are operating.

Use of the National Monitoring Checklist
The national monitoring checklist developed by the MOPH is used in MOPH–SM provinces and provinces covered by USAID. It is also used in some provinces supported by the European Commission and the MOPH, and preparations are under way to implement it in the remaining provinces.

Coordination of Development Partners

Better coordination of development partners requires both a focus on results and tighter coordination at the provincial level. This section examines both issues.

Results Focus
The level of coordination in the sector is weak on results and needs strengthening. For example, the MOPH has no clear view of all the various kinds of technical assistance provided by different donors in the sector.[5]

A number of committees and forums have been set up to ensure functional coordination. At the central level, these include the NTCC, the CGHN, the TAG, and the BPHS.[6] Findings from the Balanced Score Card, HMIS reports, NGO quarterly reports, surveys, and research projects are discussed at NTCC, BPHS, and CGHN meetings at the central level. Based on the findings, the Health Economics and Finance Directorate holds separate meetings with NGOs, develops action plans, and follows up on decisions made to address the identified problems. Some vertical programs, such as the EPI, have separate and specific coordination mechanisms at the national level.

A working CGHN, chaired by the deputy minister for technical affairs, meets weekly and serves as a venue in which to discuss and coordinate technical and policy issues. The large CGHN—which includes representatives from other ministries, donors, UN agencies, and selected NGOs—meets once a month, chaired by the MOPH. On technical issues, ad hoc task forces are established around specific issues to advise the CGHN and the TAG.

Coordination at the Provincial Level

At the provincial level, all activities, including those of vertical programs and the BPHS, are coordinated through the PHCC. The level of data use and the discussion of results at PHCC meetings vary considerably across provinces. In one province, for example, officials used the data to find that coverage of Directly Observed Therapy Short Course (DOTS) was extremely low. Based on these findings, they planned community mobilization and outreach services and continue to use routine reports to monitor progress. In another province, managers acknowledged that they rely almost entirely on direct field visits and community feedback for making decisions because of lack of trained HMIS officers and limited cooperation from the NGO. Overall, the presence of provincial advisors seems to improve the focus on results. The discussion of results varies depending on the availability of qualified HMIS officers and the cooperation of NGOs.

Information, Education, and Communication/Behavior Change Communication

The Information, Education, and Communication/Behavior Change Communication (IEC/BCC) Department of the Afghan Public Health Institute is charged with leading the ministry's healthy behavior promotion activities. The department has more than 30 nontechnical staff and

8 regional officers, who coordinate IEC activities at the regional level. The department receives support from various donors, including the Global Alliance for Vaccines and Immunization (GAVI), United Nations Children's Fund (UNICEF), and the United Nations Population Fund (UNFPA). This support is poorly coordinated, however, and the budget is underspent, reportedly because of complicated procurement and administrative procedures and lack of capacity in the department.

IEC/BCC activities suffer from a lack of clear direction. IEC is not well defined in the BPHS, and no one is specifically designated to conduct IEC activities in health facilities, which creates a disconnect between IEC and the BPHS. There is also a sense that the main sources of information, such as the Balanced Score Card and HMIS reports, do not include specific indicators for IEC.

The MOPH does not have a single coherent IEC/BCC strategy. The IEC/BCC Department has been working on IEC policy, strategy, and guidelines for more than two years. The documents are still in draft form because of a lack of technical expertise even among the international counterparts and supporting organizations. Other departments and programs of the ministry have developed their IEC documents with or without the collaboration of the IEC Department.

None of the existing documents is clear about the key messages, who should deliver them, and their resource requirements. There are two draft strategies, with the following components: maternal health, child health, EPI, nutrition, communicable diseases, and environmental health. For each component, the documents present specific objectives (in terms of health outcomes), strategies, long lists of behaviors to be changed, a detailed list of activities, and an extended list of indicators and communication channels.

In the absence of a national strategy, provinces conduct their own IEC/BCC, with little guidance. PHO officials reported that they have conducted IEC campaigns on polio, avian influenza, and salt iodization after receiving instructions from the MOPH on an ad hoc basis, with resources provided by the MOPH or UNICEF. No systematic evaluation has been carried out to evaluate the impact of these activities.

Emergency Response

The ministry has yet to establish a unified emergency preparedness and response unit. Emergency preparedness and response are dealt with by several directorates and departments in the ministry, including the DEWS Department (part of the Afghan Public Health Institute General Directorate), the Emergency Preparedness and Response (EPR) Department, the EPI Department (part of the Health Care Services Provision General Directorate), and the Provincial Health Liaison Office.

The absence of a single unit responsible for emergency response and overall guidelines for emergency preparation and response has contributed to the lack of resources. Although Afghanistan is vulnerable to numerous emergencies, no specific funds are available for emergencies other than avian influenza, the DEWS, and preparation for the winter. According to Provincial Health Liaison Office officials, provinces that are at high risk during the winter have been identified, and an action plan has been laid out, with financial support from UNICEF. The DEWS has a structured data analysis system for monitoring and in case of outbreak; the Afghan Public Health Institute contacts partners in the health sector for mobilizing resources. Some provinces have provincial emergency subcommittees to lead activities and mobilize resources locally and from the central government in case of emergencies. BPHS–implementing NGOs are also expected to assist in responding to emergencies in their respective provinces.

EPI and DEWS teams, including the control of communicable disease officers of the PHOs, are trained in outbreak response and emergency preparedness based on the WHO reference material. Provincial rapid response teams also have been trained. No field simulation has been carried out to date. With the outbreak of H1N1 in late 2009 (1388 AC), practical experience was gained that can be used in similar emergencies.

Concluding Remarks: Findings and Recommendations

Setting Strategies and Objectives

Several key findings are evident. There is no effective mechanism for disseminating policies, strategies, and guidelines to MOPH staff at the central and provincial levels. There are delays in disseminating the common list of national health indicators to stakeholders and MOPH staff. Provincial officials are not involved in the development of MOPH technical documents.

Several recommendations emerge from these findings:

- There is an urgent need to put in place a formal system for distributing MOPH key documents to MOPH departments and PHOs. Developing such a system could be attained with little effort, given that a functioning Provincial Health Liaison Office exists, documents are available in the MOPH Resource Center, and PHO staff visit the MOPH regularly.

- The MOPH should consider reinitiating the quarterly provincial health workshops for keeping provincial health directors up to date on new developments in the MOPH; giving them feedback on their performance; explaining new policies and strategies; presenting the HMIS, Balanced Score Card, and survey and research findings; answering questions; and giving provincial health directors an opportunity to share their comments and experiences.

- Involving the PHOs in the development and revision of policies and strategies could be extremely useful. As PHOs cannot attend task force meetings weekly, this could be achieved by making several provinces members of a task force or working group and asking the provinces to attend the meetings by turns.

- Finalizing and publishing the list of national health indicators and producing provincial factsheets, as envisaged in the draft M&E strategic plan, would sharpen the focus on results.

Budget and Resource Mobilization

Several key findings are evident. There is no designated operational budget for departments or PHOs, which have no involvement in budget preparation. Reform of the GDA has been delayed, administrative and procurement procedures are outdated, there are delays in processing Mostofiats, financial authority is centralized and delegation lacking, and there is no strategy for resource mobilization.

Several recommendations emerge from these findings:

- Managers in the MOPH and PHOs should have greater involvement in the budget process, knowledge of their budgets, and a gradually increasing amount of control over expenditure decisions. The Ministry of Finance program budgeting pilot in some ministries, including the MOPH, should be used as an opportunity to allow managers to develop, control, and execute their budgets at the central and provincial levels. This opportunity should also be used to separate the budgets of PHOs from the budgets of hospitals.

- Decentralization of the budget and financial authority should be accompanied by decentralizing decision making and empowering MOPH departments and PHOs. Doing so would not only bring realities on the ground closer to decision making, rendering the entire system more efficient and effective, it would also free up more time for senior MOPH officials to focus on more strategic issues.

- Channeling funds to provinces through private banks could be explored to address the problem of delays in releasing funds and other administrative bottlenecks at the Mostofiats.

- The MOPH should encourage directorates and PHOs to mobilize resources, provide them with guidelines on doing so, and enhance their negotiation and proposal-writing skills.

Monitoring and Evaluation and Use of Data

Several key findings are evident. Knowledge of indicators of success is lacking, and the use of data for decision making at the central and provincial levels is inconsistent. There is no regular preparation and dissemination of a list of national health indicators or provincial summary sheets. There is a shortage of qualified HMIS officers at the provincial level. The Balanced Score Card is an important tool, but it is not put to optimal use, because the timing of the surveys at individual health facilities is too predictable, there are potential conflicts of interest on the part of data collectors, there is a prolonged gap between data collection and the preparation of the report, and the level of sophistication of the Balanced Score Card makes it difficult to understand and use as a management tool.

Three recommendations emerge from these findings:

- The MOPH should finalize a factsheet for summarizing data from various sources—including HMIS and quarterly reports, similar to the Balanced Score Card—in order to give managers a snapshot of health system performance across the country and provinces each quarter. The report could also be published on the MOPH Web site. The summary, along with the feedback, could be communicated to the provinces.

- The MOPH and its partners may want to explore ways to improve the Balanced Score Card. Options to consider include making it entirely independent, with data collection carried out by independent data collectors who are not associated with the NGOs or PHOs; using the

M&E staff of the MOPH to conduct quality control for data collection and compilation; and conducting surveys according to a schedule not known in advance by facilities.

- The MOPH should assess the level of knowledge and the extent of use of the Balanced Score Card and the HMIS in the MOPH and PHOs and conduct appropriate training to fill gaps. It would also be helpful to make better use of the Balanced Score Card database and background information at the provincial level.

Accountability and Responsiveness

Several key findings are evident. Access to the MOPH Web site is constrained by the fact that it is available only in English and provides only a limited range of information. Policies and guidelines about information sharing and public relations are lacking.

Improving public relations requires more staff and investments, including Web designers, translators, and IT equipment, as well as guidelines and instructions for MOPH departments and PHOs regarding their public relations and accountability obligations. This should be possible with available financial resources. The MOPH already has a draft public relations strategy, which if revised, could serve as the basis for developing a more comprehensive one.

Technical Guidelines and Supervision

Several key findings are evident. There are no technical guidelines for the mental health, disability, and IEC components of the BPHS and no standard treatment guidelines for the EPHS. There is no effective mechanism for distributing technical guidelines to the MOPH and PHO staff. There are inconsistencies in the training of PHO staff on technical guidelines and in the use of the national monitoring checklist by the MOPH and PHO officials. Supervision of the PHOs is limited.

Three recommendations emerge from these findings:

- Guidelines for the mental health, disability, and IEC parts of the BPHS and standard treatment guidelines for the EPHS should be developed.
- The MOPH can conduct consistent training in all PHOs on guidelines, policies, strategies, technical guidelines, the national monitoring checklist, the HMIS, and the Balanced Score Card.
- It would be helpful to develop a supervisory checklist for the PHOs and to institute regular supervision of them.

Coordination of Development Partners

Several key findings are evident. Coordination meetings at the central and provincial levels are not uniform. They vary in the ways in which they present results, discuss findings, base decision making on data, and follow up.

Two recommendations emerge from these findings:

- Presentation of findings based on the selected indicators, discussion, decision making, and follow-up should all become integral parts of all coordination meeting agendas.
- The MOPH should make sure that NGOs submit their activity reports to the PHOs. This can be achieved, for example, by requiring NGOs to obtain the signature of a PHO official on their reports certifying that the official has been given a copy of the report.

IEC/BCC

Several key findings are evident. There is a shortage of technical staff and technical expertise in the IEC/BCC Department. There has been a delay in the finalization of the IEC/BCC strategies and guidelines. The IEC/BCC Department is isolated from the health care delivery departments of the ministry.

Two recommendations emerge from these findings:

- A short-term IEC/BCC specialist should be hired to accelerate completion of policies, strategies, guidelines, and a national plan.
- The IEC/BCC Department should be integrated with health care delivery departments by moving it into the General Directorate of Health Services Provision and involving it in BPHS coordination meetings.

Emergency Response

Several key findings are evident. No national plan or guidelines for emergencies exist. There is no preparation for certain types of emergencies. Emergency response functions are fragmented among several directorates.

Four recommendations emerge from these findings:

- The MOPH should integrate the departments that deal with emergencies under a single umbrella. In particular, strengthening the Emergency Preparedness and Response Unit is critical.

- The Emergency Preparedness and Response Unit should prepare general guidelines and instructions for PHOs and MOPH departments.
- The MOPH should conduct an annual or perhaps a semiannual assessment of potential sources of emergencies and map the resources at the central and provincial levels.
- The MOPH should ensure that the emergency subcommittees in all provinces are functioning.

Notes

1. The CGHN includes major stakeholders in health, including donors, UN agencies, and representatives of NGOs.
2. Technical Support to the Central and Provincial Ministry of Public Health (Tech-Serve) Project works with the Ministry of Public Health (MOPH) at the central and provincial levels to build its capacity to perform its primary function of guiding the health system by establishing national health objectives that address national health priorities while ensuring equity and fostering sustainability.
3. This process involves appraising civil servants to determine whether they qualify for a higher level of payment.
4. PHCC meetings are held monthly in each province. They are attended by the staff of the concerned PHO, NGOs, the World Health Organization (WHO), UNICEF, and other health stakeholders.
5. The ministry is trying to map all technical assistance provided by donors.
6. BPHS coordination meetings are attended by BPHS NGOs and chaired by the GDPP.

CHAPTER 8

Concluding Remarks: Moving Forward

Afghanistan has made considerable progress since 2003 (1382 AC), but much remains to be done. Service coverage has expanded dramatically, resulting in increases in antenatal care, skilled birth attendance, and vaccination coverage. This increase in coverage has contributed to the reduction in maternal and child mortality. Despite this progress, however, Afghanistan continues to have some of the poorest health outcomes in the world. The child mortality rate and maternal mortality ratio still remain among the world's highest. Coverage of some essential health services remains well below that of neighboring countries.

As rightly stressed in the health and nutrition sector strategy, further expanding the coverage of the basic package of health services (BPHS) should be a priority; the package of services in the BPHS should be expanded only judiciously. Currently, about 60 percent of Afghanistan's population lives more than an hour's walking distance from a health facility. Reducing this distance to the level stated in the health and nutrition sector strategy would significantly increase service coverage. The Ministry of Public Health (MOPH) can draw on its own successful experience in expanding coverage under difficult circumstances. Expansion of the scope of services in the BPHS should not take priority over expanding coverage.

Any expansion of the package should be viewed against the opportunity cost it entails in terms of expanding its coverage.

Expanding coverage requires more resource mobilization and improved budget execution. Although what to do in order to expand coverage is clear, the means to do so present significant challenges. The flattening of external assistance to the sector has increased pressure on resources. The MOPH should focus on both mobilizing additional resources and improving its spending ability.

The MOPH could better leverage the private sector to complement its effort to expand BPHS coverage and improve quality. The private sector is providing services to a large segment of the population in rural Afghanistan. The ministry could partner with physicians in solo practice, who dominate the private sector in rural Afghanistan, to expand services. Such arrangements could be attractive for expanding services in insecure areas that are beyond the reach of NGOs.

The MOPH needs to address the human resource shortage and imbalances in the public sector. A number of short- and long-term options could address these problems. In the short term, the MOPH could consider hiring health workers on a contractual basis, with renewal of contracts made conditional on performance. In the long term, the MOPH will need to address the imbalances in the health workforce by giving female workers and people working in remote areas preferential treatment for training opportunities and other incentives.

Finally, building the institutional capacity of the ministry is critical to expanding the BPHS further, better mobilizing resources, and partnering with the private sector. It is also essential in addressing the human resource problems the sector is facing.

Specific Recommendations

In what follows, specific policy options are presented for the MOPH to consider to build on the early gains it has made in the health sector. The guiding principles of these options are consistent with the ministry's vision and feasibility. For ease of reference, the options are presented for the issues covered in each chapter of this book; they should be taken together, as part of overall guidance for the sector. These policy options tell a story, the central theme of which is the need to expand service coverage and what the ministry needs to do to make that happen.

The section starts with options to expand coverage. It then identifies options for mobilizing financial resources to pay for the expansion, reviews options for harnessing the private sector to expand coverage, and looks at how human resource problems can be addressed to enable service expansion. It closes with suggestions for building the institutional capacity of the ministry to enable it to perform all these tasks effectively.

Strengthening the BPHS

Expanding the coverage of the BPHS is of the utmost importance. Coverage of services may be expanded through the following proven strategies:

- Expanding subcenters to reach remote areas
- Training and deploying motivated and compensated community health workers
- Critically evaluating the experiments being piloted.

Monitoring and evaluation (M&E) is important for the sustained success of the BPHS. The government should invest in continuing the collection of nonadministrative data to strengthen M&E. At a minimum, two sources of data should be maintained: household surveys every two years and annual facility surveys.

The content of the BPHS should be open for periodic revision but based on solid principles. These principles include consistency with the health and nutrition sector strategy, affordability and cost-effectiveness, equity aspects of the intervention, and ease of implementation and inclusion of the existing package without displacing other BPHS services.

Financing the Sector

More resources are needed to expand service coverage. Public financing for the health sector has increased significantly since 2003 (1382 AC), reaching $10.92 per capita in 2008 (1387 AC). This per capita expenditure still falls short of the level necessary to provide primary health care free of charge and with universal access. Expansion of service to the more remote and poorer areas in particular is heavily dependent on the availability of additional finance. The government should assess the potential for maintaining user fees for nonprimary care services, with appropriate exemptions for low-income patients, to generate resources. More resources could also potentially be mobilized through the following means:

- *Improved budgetary execution.* Improving the ministry's budget execution from its current level of 54 percent would release substantial resources with which to expand service coverage.

- *Use of Afghanistan Reconstruction Trust Fund (ARTF) and other multi-lateral and bilateral sources.* New sources of finance should be explored. The recent effort to access the ARTF is a successful example.
- *Cost-effective spending.* Carefully selecting cost-effective interventions and programs would ensure that resources are used more efficiently.

Protecting households from large out-of-pocket payments is critical. Such payments, a large share of which is spent on pharmaceuticals, constitute about 79 percent of total spending on health. The government could explore policies to reduce out-of-pocket health expenditures. For example, some form of community-based insurance in partnership with private providers could be explored.

Establishing a system of national health accounts (NHAs) is essential. An NHA would provide a useful management tool for tracking the flow of funds through the health sector, from their sources, through financial institutions, to providers and functions. The institutionalization of a system of NHAs is an area the government should focus on. The ministry should use the opportunity of growing donor interest in this area to institutionalize the NHA.

Involving the Private Sector

Private and public providers in rural Afghanistan provide largely complementary services that can be enhanced through appropriate policies that harness the energy of the private sector. Steps could include the following:

- A unit to work with the private sector should be established within the MOPH. The MOPH has begun preparing related documents and establishing a new unit, including a task force for organizing private sector–related activities, which are scattered across different departments. The urgency of acting on this front has been recognized. This volume should help guide the initial stages of the unit's engagement with the private sector.

- Parallel to efforts to improve the quality of care of publicly provided health services, the MOPH should work to improve the quality of service in the private sector. This could be done by encouraging the participation of private providers in quality assessment surveys along the lines of the Balanced Score Card. There are different means of encouraging the participation of private providers in quality assessments, including regulatory measures, contracting, and incentives.

The MOPH has a range of instruments at its disposal. No single instrument would provide the desired result; the optimal approach may involve a combination of instruments that are not mutually exclusive. Potential instruments include the following:

- *Regulatory controls and restrictions*. These instruments involve legal requirements to which providers must conform. Violating these restrictions would result in some kind of penalty. The effectiveness of these instruments depends on the capacity of the ministry to set standards and monitor and enforce compliance. The current inclination at the MOPH seems to favor this instrument. However, given its limited capacity to set standards and monitor and enforce compliance, the ministry should use these instruments for licensing but not for regular monitoring.
- *Incentives*. Incentives are bonus payments and penalties the ministry would develop to encourage providers to change behavior in order to achieve desired targets for quality or coverage.
- *Contracting*. The MOPH could exert significant influence over the private sector if it contracted with private providers for complementary services or to expand some services in the BPHS.
- *Information dissemination*. Information dissemination involves making information on providers available to users so that consumers can make informed decisions that encourage providers to improve service quality.

Improving Human Resources for Health
Afghanistan's health workforce suffers from three main imbalances:

- *Geographic imbalance*. The workforce is highly concentrated in urban areas.
- *Gender imbalance*. There is a shortage of female staff, especially in rural areas.
- *Skills-mix imbalance*. There is a shortage of staff with nutrition, public health, reproductive health, and child health skills.

The current draft of the human resources policy may need to be revised to better reflect a strategic vision and implementation approach to address these imbalances. The human resources for health strategy and policy need to translate the guiding principles into a coherent action plan for addressing the human resource imbalance in the country. The action plan should specify the responsibilities of various actors, the resource requirements, and the timeframe for implementation. In the short term, training community midwives and nurses must form the cornerstone of such a plan.

Suggested steps to address the human resource imbalances include the following:

- *Incentives.* The government should create incentives to make working in the health sector more attractive for women and people willing to work in remote areas. The government retains near monopoly power over the medical education system. It could, for example, grant preferential admission for women and people committing to work in remote areas. It is also possible to make postings to attractive locations conditional on first filling a commitment to work in a remote area. This approach is used in Bangladesh, where points are awarded for working in remote areas and accumulation of points increases the likelihood of future postings in more attractive locations.

- *Professional development.* The data show that health workers are unlikely to find opportunities for professional development once they leave Kabul. Making professional development opportunities available to staff working in more remote areas may provide incentives for working in these locations, which would in turn improve the quality of the health workforce.

An important aspect of the human resources strategy should include piloting approaches to hiring and compensation that motivate good performance. Examples include the following:

- *Relating payments/benefits to place of work and performance.* A proposed experiment, through the results-based financing pilot, to motivate health workers through additional payment linked to performance would provide new sets of evidence on the possibility of using such a mechanism to recruit and retain workers in remote areas.

- *Hiring health facility staff on a contract basis.* This strategy would be useful for a number of reasons. First, it would help the MOPH avoid any long-term contingent liabilities that hiring permanent employees implies. Given that about half of the current budget goes to staff salary and benefits, this could be an attractive alternative to the MOPH.

Second, it would increase managers' ability to ensure that staff focus on performance. Third, it would allow flexible remuneration, which would be a useful instrument for promptly responding to emerging human resource problems. Contractual hiring could also be a broader intervention than salary increases for attracting and retaining female health workers in remote areas.

Strengthening the Institutional Capacity of the Ministry

There are a number of areas in which the ministry should strengthen its capacity to carry out its stewardship functions. The following areas should be given priority:

- A single unit that coordinates the various departments' work with the private sector should be established and strengthened.

- The unit responsible for resource mobilization and tracking of expenditures should be strengthened.

- Managers in the MOPH and PHOs should be involved in the budgetary process and exert a gradually increasing amount of control over expenditure decisions. The Ministry of Finance program budgeting pilot should be used as an opportunity to allow the managers to develop, control, and execute their budgets at the central and provincial levels. This opportunity should also be used for separating the budgets of the PHOs from the budgets of the hospitals. The ministry should develop a clear information, education, and communication/behavior change communication (IEC/BCC) strategy before capacity building in this area is considered.

- In addition to strengthening the units in its headquarters in Kabul, the ministry should use the immense potential of its provincial offices to broaden its stewardship role. The PHOs could be given a larger role in a number of areas, including supervising the implementing NGOs, coordinating the activities of various stakeholders at the provincial level, promoting IEC/BCC activities, and working with the for-profit private sector, including on regulation.

Domains and Components of the Balanced Score Card

Table A.1 Domains and Components of the Balanced Score Card

Domain	Component
Patients and community	• Overall patient satisfaction
	• Patient perceptions of quality
	• *Shura-e-sehie* (community health committee) active in community
Staff	• Health worker satisfaction
	• Salary payments current
Capacity for service provision	• Equipment functionality
	• Drug availability
	• Family planning availability
	• Laboratory functionality
	• Staffing levels
	• Provider knowledge score
	• Staff training in past year
	• Use of Health Management Information System (HMIS)
	• Clinical guidelines
	• Infrastructure
	• Patient record keeping
	• Monitoring of tuberculosis treatment

(continued)

Table A.1   *(continued)*

Domain	Component
Service provision	• Patient history and physical exam • Patient counseling • Proper disposal of sharps • Average number of new outpatient visits per month exceeds 750 per basic health center • More than nine minutes spent with each patient • Provision of antenatal care • Provision of delivery care
Financial systems	• User fee guidelines at facilities • Exemptions for poor patients at facilities
MOPH vision	• Equity of service delivery • Equity of patient satisfaction • Females as percentage of new outpatients

Source: Author.

Data Collection Issues and Presentation

Data availability is always constrained by the reporting requirements of the government and various donors and by constraints imposed by economic actors. For example, because of the flexible budgetary approach used in Ministry of Public Health (MOPH)/World Bank basic package of health services (BPHS) contracts, no detailed financial reports were available from the implementing nongovernmental organizations (NGOs). This is a different approach from that taken by the European Commission. Similarly, as the essential package of health services (EPHS) and the BPHS are contracted as a single package by the European Commission, no breakdown of cost by line of activity was available.

Data Analysis and Presentation

Data are presented for Afghan calendar (AC) years (see appendix C) in order to avoid discrepancies with the national budget cycle. As all programs started at different dates, each line of assistance was recomputed to correspond with the Afghan year. For external assistance, estimation of financing was based on money actually spent in Afghanistan, not money disbursed by headquarters (when it was possible to identify them, headquarters' management costs were also calculated). Completed contracts and programs were taken at their actual value (based on financial execution reports when available). For uncompleted contracts and programs for 2008 (1387 AC), estimations were based on the expenditure rate since the beginning of the contract or program and the total and remaining budget. The rate of implementation was determined by comparing the initial budget with the actual expenditure and the initial completion date with the actual completion date or extension requested.

Exchange Rate

Data were collected in the currency of the donor agency. Funds obtained in foreign currency were converted into U.S. dollars using the average annual rate of exchange of the period under consideration from the Oanda Web site (http://www.oanda.com/convert/fxhistory).

Population Data

Lack of accurate and recent census data is a well-known problem in Afghanistan. As best estimates, this study used household listings from the Central Statistics Office. The listing was done between 2002 (1381 AC) and 2005 (1384 AC) in preparation for the Afghan census.

Data on Type, Activity, Area, and Program

Type/activity refers to the major activities undertaken by agencies and programs, such as training, capacity building, technical assistance to the MOPH, health care delivery (such as the BPHS and EPHS), monitoring and evaluation, studies, infrastructure and equipment, procurement and supplies, and administration and management. When data on expenditures per activity were missing or the majority of activities were classified as "general" or "operations," expenditures were allocated as per the general mandate of the organization. For example, in the case of UN technical agencies (the World Health Organization, the United Nations Population Fund [UNFPA], United Nations Children's Fund [UNICEF]), expenditures were classified mainly under "technical assistance," unless otherwise specified (as in the case of procurement of vaccines by UNICEF, for example).

Area/program refers to broad areas of priority, such as disease programs (reproductive health, nutrition, tuberculosis, malaria, HIV/AIDS, disability, the Expanded Program on Immunization [EPI], and so forth) and functional areas (primary health care, hospitals, health system support, and so forth). The definition of programs corresponds as closely as possible to the MOPH program categories used for program budgeting, based on the health care strategy of the Afghanistan national development strategy.

Limitations and Challenges

In the absence of national health accounts, data collection was a major challenge that took a disproportionate share of the time allocated for the study. Several bilateral donors that had been involved in the health sector in 2002–03 (1381–82 AC) but were no longer funding health programs could not provide any information. For some donors, data on closed projects had to be retrieved from headquarters. Retrieval of information from donors' systems was a labor-intensive process that involved, in some cases, reviewing each contract over the five-year study period. For all donors and agencies, data collection required numerous meetings, calls, and follow-up contacts.

Financial information on construction was not always accessible: data on most civil and military construction programs supported by the United States (by far the most active country in this domain) were available, but data on other Provincial Reconstruction Team and some bilateral construction aid (from Brunei, China, and Turkey) were not.[1] The decentralized nature of many activities (Provincial Reconstruction Team projects as well as small projects implemented by NGOs with bilateral support) made data collection difficult, as no information was available at the central level. The International Relations Department of the MOPH collects and keeps the Memoranda of Understanding signed by the donors and the government, but no data were obtained from it.

When it was not possible to rely on direct data collection from donors, some information was sourced from the Ministry of Finance Aid Coordination database. This database is not exhaustive (notably for 2006/07–2008/09 [1385–87 AC]); in most cases it contain figures only on commitments, not disbursements; and it contains redundancies and inaccuracies, uncovered by cross-checking with donors. Double counting is widespread, which leads to substantial overestimation of external funding. For example, UN technical agency funding and bilateral funding were often counted twice (examples include immunization under UNICEF and bilateral agencies and some disease programs under the World Health Organization and bilateral agencies), and some bilateral aid was counted under two different programs.

Within the MOPH, operating budget data were obtained from the Finance and Administration Directorate, but this unit is not computerized and each request had to be manually processed, taking at least a week after translation from Dari into English. In contrast, budget and treasury data were available on the Ministry of Finance's Web site; this transparency is commendable. Budget documents and decrees are comprehensive and well presented. However, reliable budget and expenditure data were available only for 2005/06–2008/09 (1384–87 AC).

Methodological Challenges

The lack of comparability of data across programs and donors was a major challenge. For example, the BPHS perimeter varies in time and across donors, in the following ways:

- The European Commission combines the EPHS and the BPHS in the same contracts, as does the U.S. Agency for International Development (USAID) under the REACH project, which operated from 2004 to 2006 (1383 AC–1385 AC). It was not possible to disaggregate the two activities, even working with the contracted NGOs, which do not maintain separate accounting.
- Training, capacity building, and drug procurement are included in the contracts of the World Bank and the European Commission but provided separately under USAID contracts.
- Construction costs were included in the early BPHS contracts with the European Commission but not in contracts with the World Bank or USAID.
- The "districts cluster" approach of the first generation of BPHS contracts made the evaluation and comparison of expenditures difficult in some provinces.

Categorization of expenditure was difficult in some cases, for the following reasons:

- Some expenditures (for training, supplies, and some construction, for example) included in the BPHS were allocated to "health care delivery" under primary health care. The rules governing the allocation of costs between technical assistance and training as well as between capacity building and management costs are unclear.
- Some categories used by donors do not correspond to MOPH programs (such as mother and child health) or cover several programs.
- Social marketing is difficult to allocate. The MOPH decided to classify it under maternal and child health, given its major focus on contraception, family health, and oral rehydration salts.
- Some programs consist largely of technical assistance but include a variable proportion of supplies (for example, procurement of zinc supplement under a program funded by USAID).

- Classification by programs inevitably underestimates cross-contributions (examples of such spillover effects include primary health care, reproductive health, EPI, and the treatment and prevention of tuberculosis).
- Geographical disaggregation was very difficult in most cases, except for clearly provincial targeted expenditure such as the BPHS and EPHS.

Note

1. By the end of 2004 (1383 AC), there were 19 Provincial Reconstruction Teams, each operating differently, reflecting national approaches. The difficulties of developing a common approach stem from the large number of countries involved, the presence of two separate military operations and commands (International Security Assistance Force (ISAF)/North Atlantic Treaty Organization (NATO) and the Combined Forces Command), and different approaches to civil and military activities (Hendrickson and others 2005).

APPENDIX C

Afghan Calendar

Table C.1   Afghan Calendar

Afghan year	Gregorian calendar period
1382	March 21, 2003–March 20, 2004
1383	March 21, 2004–March 20, 2005
1384	March 21, 2005–March 20, 2006
1385	March 21, 2006–March 20, 2007
1386	March 21, 2007–March 20, 2008
1387	March 21, 2008–March 20, 2009

Survey of Private Health Providers

A survey was designed to fill the gap in information about the private sector and better understand the private sector in rural Afghanistan. The focus was on identifying the type and mix of private providers in rural communities, patterns of household utilization, and quality and service capacity.

Survey Design and Sampling

In the absence of a comprehensive registry or sampling frame for private providers, an alternative method was used by which the household survey was linked to the provider survey. The survey consisted of linked samples of households and providers, to ensure that it adequately represented the local configuration of private health care providers used by households in rural Afghanistan. The universe of providers was generated after the return of the household survey.

Households were randomly selected from 28 villages in 14 districts and 5 provinces. A total of 776 households were selected. The survey included separate concurrent interviews with the head of the household and a woman in the household. The head of household interview focused on securing detailed information on household members and the conditions in which they live in order to provide an overview of household health care system utilization, health care access issues, and experiences in encounters with private and public sector providers. The interviews with women focused on maternal and child health issues. A provider survey of 152 private health care providers identified by the households was also conducted.

Provinces and Districts Covered

The survey covered five diverse provinces representing various parts of the country: Badghis in the northwest, Baghlan in the north, Laghman in the east, Logar in the central region, and Nimroz in the south. Within the 5 provinces, 14 rural districts were selected from two strata of districts. One stratum comprises densely populated districts. It includes the central districts in which provincial capitals are located but not the capital city itself. The other stratum includes all other districts in the province. This stratum represents rural districts, where access to health care is generally more difficult and coverage of health care lower. In each of the provinces, three districts were selected: two from rural districts and one from the central district.[1]

Villages and Households Covered

In each district, two nonadjacent villages that are within three hours' (one-way) walking distance from the provincial capital were randomly selected. When a village was found to be inaccessible because of lack of security, a replacement was selected. Villages were mapped into four quadrants with two "distance rings" forming eight areas (an "inner" and an "outer" ring in each of the four quadrants [northeast, southeast, southwest, northwest]). A total of 28 households were selected from each of the eight areas of the village.

Given the heterogeneity of households within a village, the design allowed for a fair number of households within a village to capture ethnic, language, and tribal diversity. The minimum size for a village to be sampled was 50 households, so that no more than 50 percent of the households were selected. In total, 787 households were selected, of which 778 were interviewed. Within those households, 667 women were interviewed.

Private Providers Covered

The initial design was to interview all private providers identified at the village level who provided health care services within the 15 sample districts. Doing so proved impossible. In particular, covering providers located outside the province was challenging.[2] A total of 152 private providers were surveyed.

Household Profile

The survey was conducted in the central district of each of the five provinces (except Logar) and in two randomly chosen rural districts of each province. Thus, about twice as many households were surveyed in the rural districts as in the central districts of the sample provinces. The survey in the central district of Logar was suspended because of security risks to the field staff. Details of demographic, education, income, and other socioeconomic profiles of the households surveyed are given in tables D1–D12.

Table D.1   Percentage and Number of Households Interviewed, by Province

Province	Total	Central district	Rural district
Badghis	21.6 (168)	33.3 (56)	66.7 (112)
Baghlan	21.3 (165)	33.3 (55)	66.7 (110)
Laghman	21.4 (166)	33.7 (56)	66.3 (110)
Logar	14.2 (110)	0	100.0 (110)
Nimroz	21.5 (167)	33.5 (56)	66.5 (111)
Total	100.0 (776)	28.7 (223)	71.3 (553)

Source: Author.
Note: Figures are percentage of all households in province interviewed; figures in parentheses are actual number of households interviewed.

Table D.2   Size Distribution of Households

Household size	Percentage and number of households
2	2.1 (16)
3	2.5 (19)
4	6.7 (51)
5	10.7 (81)
6	14.2 (107)
7	16.7 (126)
8	13.5 (102)
9	11.0 (83)
10	8.2 (62)
10+	14.4 (109)
Total	100.0 (756)

Source: Author.
Note: Figures are percentage of all households of each size interviewed; figures in parentheses are actual number of households of each size.

Table D.3   Age Distribution, by Gender

Age group	Male	Female	Total	Male/female gender ratio
0–4	47.9 (323)	52.1 (352)	12.5 (675)	0.92
5–9	52.4 (454)	47.6 (413)	16.1 (867)	1.10
10–14	52.8 (427)	47.2 (381)	15.0 (808)	1.12
15–19	56.6 (357)	43.4 (274)	11.7 (631)	1.30
20–24	60.6 (251)	39.4 (163)	7.7 (414)	1.54
25–29	57.2 (198)	42.8 (148)	6.4 (346)	1.34
30–34	52.2 (154)	47.8 (141)	5.5 (295)	1.09
35–39	51.0 (146)	49.0 (140)	5.3 (286)	1.04
40–44	54.1 (138)	45.9 (117)	4.7 (255)	1.18
45–49	55.2 (116)	44.8 (94)	3.9 (210)	1.23
50–54	56.3 (94)	43.7 (73)	3.1 (167)	1.29
55–59	71.6 (68)	28.4 (27)	1.8 (95)	2.52
60–64	64.0 (80)	36.0 (45)	2.3 (125)	1.78
65+	73.0 (154)	27.0 (57)	3.9 (211)	2.70
Total	55.0 (2,960)	45.0 (2,425)	100 (5,385)	1.22

Source: Author.
Note: Figures are percentage of all men and women in each age group interviewed; figures in parentheses are actual number of households interviewed.

Table D.4   Average Age and Education of Household Head
(years)

Region	Average age	Average education
Badghis	48.6	2.6
Central	49.1	4.0
Rural	48.4	1.9
Baghlan	48.1	2.7
Central	48.8	2.7
Rural	47.7	2.7
Laghman	42.6	5.3
Central	46.5	6.8
Rural	40.5	4.6
Logar	48.1	6.5
Nimroz	44.4	1.6
Central	43.8	1.6
Rural	44.7	1.6
Total	46.2	3.5
Central	47.1	3.8
Rural	45.9	3.4

Source: Author.

Table D.5 School Attendance, by Age Group and Gender

Age group (years)	Male		Female		Total		
	Never attended	Attended	Never attended	Attended	Never attended	Attended	Total
5–9	53.3 (235)	46.7 (206)	61.3 (247)	38.7 (156)	57.1 (482)	42.9 (362)	844
10–14	22.6 (96)	77.4 (328)	48.7 (182)	51.3 (192)	34.8 (278)	65.2 (520)	798
15–19	35.1 (124)	64.9 (229)	68.0 (185)	32.0 (87)	49.4 (309)	50.6 (316)	625
20–24	43.2 (108)	56.8 (142)	89.9 (143)	10.1 (16)	61.4 (251)	38.6 (158)	409
25–29	45.5 (89)	54.6 (107)	90.4 (132)	9.6 (14)	64.6 (221)	35.4 (121)	342
30–34	56.2 (86)	43.8 (67)	97.9 (137)	2.1 (3)	76.1 (223)	23.9 (70)	293
35–39	50.0 (73)	50.0 (73)	94.1 (128)	5.9 (8)	71.3 (201)	28.7 (81)	282
40–44	54.3 (75)	45.7 (63)	91.3 (105)	8.7 (10)	71.1 (180)	28.9 (73)	253
45–49	47.4 (55)	52.6 (61)	98.9 (89)	1.1 (1)	69.9 (144)	30.1 (62)	206
50–54	58.7 (54)	41.3 (38)	97.1 (68)	2.9 (2)	75.3 (122)	24.7 (40)	162
55–59	68.7 (46)	31.3 (21)	100.0 (27)	0.0 (0)	77.7 (73)	22.3 (21)	94
60–64	78.5 (62)	21.5 (17)	95.6 (43)	4.4 (2)	84.7 (105)	15.3 (19)	124
65+	76.8 (116)	23.2 (35)	93.0 (53)	7.0 (4)	81.3 (169)	18.8 (39)	208
Total	46.8 (1,219)	53.2 (1,387)	75.7 (1,539)	24.3 (495)	59.4 (2,758)	40.6 (1,882)	4,640

Source: Author.

Note: Figures are percentage of all people in interviewed households by age group; figures in parentheses are actual number of people in interviewed households by age group.

Table D.6 Primary Source of Household Income

Province	Agriculture	Rearing of animals	Other labor	Business/ trading	Service professional, technical, and salaried work	Remittances	Other	Total
Badghis	82.3 (135)	7.3 (12)	3.0 (5)	1.8 (3)	1.8 (3)	0	3.7 (6)	100 (164)
Central	90.6(48)	5.7 (3)	–0	1.9 (1)	1.9 (1)	0	0	100 (53)
Rural	78.4 (87)	8.1 (9)	4.5 (5)	1.8 (2)	1.8 (2)	0	5.4 (6)	100 (111)
Baghlan	65.0 (106)	1.8 (3)	20.2 (33)	0.6 (1)	6.1 (10)	0.6 (1)	5.5 (9)	100 (163)
Central	72.2 (39)	3.7 (2)	7.4 (4)	0	9.3 (5)	0	7.4 (4)	100 (54)
Rural	61.5 (67)	0.9 (1)	26.6 (29)	0.9 (1)	4.6 (5)	0.9 (1)	4.6 (5)	100 (109)
Laghman	50.6 (83)	1.2 (2)	9.8(16)	6.1 (10)	11.6 (19)	6.1 (10)	14.6 (24)	100 (164)
Central	37.0 (20)	1.9 (1)	7.4 (4)	7.4 (4)	22.2 (12)	1.9 (1)	22.2 (12)	100 (54)
Rural	57.3 (63)	0.9 (1)	10.9 (12)	5.5(6)	6.4(7)	8.2 (9)	10.9 (12)	100 (110)
Logar	50.0 (55)	4.5 (5)	13.6 (15)	19.1 (21)	9.1 (10)	0.9 (1)	2.7 (3)	100 (110)
Nimroz	20.4 (34)	7.2 (12)	38.9 (65)	5.4(9)	24.6 (41)	0	3.6 (6)	100 (167)
Central	0	3.6 (2)	44.6 (25)	10.7 (6)	37.5 (21)	0	3.6 (2)	100 (56)
Rural	30.6 (34)	9.0 (10)	36.0 (40)	2.7 (3)	18.0 (20)	0	3.6 (4)	100 (111)
Total	53.8 (413)	4.4 (34)	17.4 (134)	5.7 (44)	10.8 (83)	1.6 (12)	6.3 (48)	100 (768)
Central	49.3 (107)	3.7 (8)	15.2 (33)	5.1 (11)	18.0 (39)	0.5 (1)	8.3 (18)	100 (217)
Rural	55.5 (306)	4.7 (26)	18.3 (101)	6.0 (33)	8.0 (44)	2.0 (11)	5.4 (30)	100 (551)

Source: Author.

Note: Figures are percentages of all households interviewed; figures in parentheses are actual number of households interviewed.

Table D.7   Ownership of Various Household Possessions, by Stratum

Possession	Central households	Rural households	Total households
Clock/watch	81.6 (182)	81.6 (451)	81.6 (633)
Pressure cooker	76.2 (170)	67.5 (373)	70.0 (543)
Sewing machine	63.2 (141)	58.8 (325)	60.1 (466)
Electric generator	17.9 (40)	8.8 (43)	10.7 (83)
Refrigerator	7.6 (17)	1.1 (6)	3.0 (23)

Source: Author.
Note: Figures are percentages of all households interviewed; figures in parentheses are actual number of households interviewed.

Table D.8   Wealth Distribution, by Province and Stratum

Province/ stratum	First quintile (poorest)	Second quintile	Third quintile	Fourth quintile	Fifth quintile (wealthiest)	Total
Badghis	20.3 (30)	29.1 (43)	27.7 (41)	17.6 (26)	5.4 (8)	148
Central	3.9 (2)	25.5 (13)	35.3 (18)	27.5 (14)	7.8 (4)	51
Rural	28.9 (28)	30.9 (30)	23.7 (23)	12.4 (12)	4.1 (4)	97
Baghlan	25.3 (38)	26.0 (39)	20.7 (31)	16.0 (24)	12.0 (18)	150
Central	18.4 (9)	18.4 (9)	24.5 (12)	20.4 (10)	18.4 (9)	49
Rural	28.7 (29)	29.7 (30)	18.8 (19)	13.9 (14)	8.9 (9)	101
Laghman	19.2 (29)	19.9 (30)	19.9 (30)	18.5 (28)	22.5 (34)	151
Central	14.0 (7)	4.0 (2)	16.0 (8)	26.0 (13)	40.0 (20)	50
Rural	21.8 (22)	27.7 (28)	21.8 (22)	14.9 (15)	13.9 (14)	101
Logar	3.7 (4)	1.9 (2)	11.1 (12)	26.9 (29)	56.5 (61)	108
Nimroz	26.7 (40)	22.0 (33)	16.7 (25)	21.3 (32)	13.3 (20)	150
Central	19.2 (10)	17.3 (9)	15.4 (8)	25.0 (13)	23.1 (12)	52
Rural	30.6·(30)	24.5 (24)	17.3 (17)	19.4 (19)	8.2 (8)	98
Total	19.9 (141)	20.8 (147)	19.7 (139)	19.7 (139)	19.9 (141)	707
Central	13.9 (28)	16.3 (33)	22.8 (46)	24.8 (50)	22.3 (45)	202
Rural	22.4 (113)	22.6 (114)	18.4 (93)	17.6 (89)	19.0 (96)	505

Source: Author.
Note: Figures are percentages of all households interviewed; figures in parentheses are actual number of households interviewed.

Table D.9 Sources of Household Water, by Province and Stratum

(percentage of all households, except where otherwise indicated)

Province/ stratum	Water sources generally considered safe						Water sources generally considered unsafe				
	Piped into household	Rainwater	Tanker or truck	Public handpump or tap	Covered well in compound	Covered well elsewhere	Open well in compound	Open well elsewhere	River, stream, pond, lake, or dam	Other	Total number of households reporting
Badghis	17.8	1.8	1.2	4.3	1.2	11.0	1.8	2.5	65.6	0	163
Central	50.0	0	0	12.5	1.8	21.4	1.8	5.4	14.3	0	56
Rural	0.9	2.8	1.9	0	0.9	5.6	1.9	0.9	92.5	0	107
Baghlan	3.0	0.6	0	26.1	7.9	10.3	10.9	5.5	44.8	1.8	165
Central	1.8	1.8	0	23.6	20.0	21.8	20.0	16.4	18.2	0.0	55
Rural	3.6	0.0	0	27.3	1.8	4.5	6.4	0.0	58.2	2.7	110
Laghman	1.2	0.6	0.6	15.3	31.9	27.6	11.0	11.7	23.3	0.6	163
Central	3.6	1.8	1.8	17.9	51.8	23.2	10.7	3.6	8.9	0	56
Rural	0	0	0	14.0	21.5	29.9	11.2	15.9	30.8	0.9	107
Logar	2.7	0	0	56.4	25.5	10.9	2.7	2.7	8.2	0	110
Nimroz	3.6	0.6	31.3	19.3	7.8	28.9	3.0	25.9	0.6	0	166
Central	10.9	1.8	90.9	5.5	5.5	1.8	3.6	5.5	0	0	55
Rural	0	0	1.8	26.1	9.0	42.3	2.7	36.0	0.9	0	111
Total	5.9	0.8	7.2	22.0	14.1	18.3	6.1	10.2	29.9	0.5	767
Central	16.7	1.4	23.0	14.9	19.8	17.1	9.0	7.7	10.4	0	222
Rural	1.5	0.6	0.7	25.0	11.7	18.7	5.0	11.2	37.8	0.7	545

Source: Author.

Table D.10   Main Household Toilet Facility, by Province
(percent, except where otherwise indicated)

Province	Field/ outside house	Traditional pit	Ordinary vault latrine	Improved vault latrine	Flush toilet	Other	Number of households
Badghis	22.7	11.7	61.7	3.9	0	0	154
Baghlan	16.3	14.4	67.5	0	0.6	1.3	160
Laghman	16.0	6.2	76.5	0	1.2	0	162
Logar	0	0	98.2	1.8	0.0	0	109
Nimroz	15.1	27.6	49.3	2.6	5.3	0	152
Total	14.9	12.6	69.1	1.6	1.5	0.3	737

Source: Author.

Table D.11   Demographics of Female Survey Respondents

Age group (years)	Number of interviews	Percentage of all interviews	Average age at marriage (years)	Average number of children
14–19	24	3.6	15.1	2.2
20–29	172	25.8	16.0	3.6
30–39	229	34.3	16.0	5.8
40–49	154	23.1	16.0	6.8
50–59	62	9.3	16.5	5.2
60–69	22	3.3	15.2	5.1
70+	4	0.6	17.3	3.5
Total	667	100	15.9	5.2

Source: Author.

Table D.12 Pregnancy Status of Female Respondents, by Age Group

Age group (years)	Pregnant at time of interview	Pregnant in current year but not now	Pregnant in last year (2007/08) (1386 AC)	Pregnant more than two years ago	Never pregnant	Will not say	Total
14–19	36.4 (8)	18.2 (4)	22.7 (5)	13.6 (3)	9.1 (2)	0 (0)	3.5 (22)
20–29	30.5 (51)	17.4 (29)	31.1 (52)	12.0 (20)	6.6 (11)	2.4 (4)	26.3 (167)
30–39	24.2 (54)	8.1 (18)	28.7 (64)	30.9 (69)	4.0 (9)	4.0 (9)	35.1 (223)
40–49	15.0 (21)	7.9 (11)	15.0 (21)	39.3 (55)	13.6 (19)	9.3 (13)	22.0 (140)
50+	4.8 (4)	6.0 (5)	2.4 (2)	53.6 (45)	14.3 (12)	19.0 (16)	13.2 (84)
Total	21.7 (138)	10.5 (67)	22.6 (144)	30.2 (192)	8.3 (53)	6.6 (42)	100 (636)

Source: Author.

Note: Figures are percentages of all individuals in age group interviewed. Figures in parentheses are actual number of individuals interviewed.

Notes

1. For security reasons, only two districts in Logar were surveyed.
2. The Baluchi in Nimroz, for instance, make extensive use of Iranian health care providers by crossing the national border.

APPENDIX E

Private Sector Health Providers

Table E.1   Types of Private Sector Health Providers Interviewed, by Province

Private sector provider	Badghis	Baghlan	Laghman	Logar	Nimroz	All five provinces
Physician	28.3 (15)	88.4 (23)	97.1 (34)	100.0 (11)	51.8 (14)	72.9 (97)
Private health clinic or hospital	0	3.8 (1)	0	0	14.8 (4)	2.2 (3)
Physician practicing in pharmacy	7.5 (4)	0	0	0	3.7 (1)	2.2 (3)
Pharmacy without physician on staff	1.9 (1)	0	0	0	11.1 (3)	1.5 (2)
Midwife and traditional birth attendant	43.4 (23)	7.7 (2)	0	0	11.1 (3)	12.8 (17)
Nurse	1.9 (1)	0	2.9 (1)	0	0	0.1 (1)
Traditional healers (including mullahs)	17.0 (9)	0	0	0	7.4 (2)	7.5 (10)
Private provider that also works in the public sector	7.5 (4)	7.8 (2)	8.6 (3)	45.5 (5)	25.9 (7)	10.5 (14)
Total	53	26	35	11	27	133

Source: Author.
Note: Figures are percentage of each type of provider out of total sampled; figures in parentheses are actual number of providers.

Human Resources for Health

According to the Ministry of Public Health (MOPH) human resources database, frontline health providers represent 48.0 percent of all human resources for health; support staff, 22.9 percent; allied health professionals and technicians, 22.6 percent; outreach workers, 3.9 percent; and managers, 2.5 percent. None of the provinces reported having a psychologist, a blood bank technician, or a nutritionist.

Table F.1   Human Resources for Health in Afghanistan, by Type of Worker

Type of provider	Number of providers
Frontline health provider	
Nurse, male	2,140
Physician, male	1,685
Midwife	1,189
Medical specialist, male	1,088
Feldsher[a]	527
Medical specialist, female	459
Nurse, female	378
Physician, female	290
Dentist	194
Anesthetist/nurse anesthetist	178
Assistant nurse, male	101
Assistant midwife	97
Assistant nurse, female	25
Subtotal	8,351
Support staff	
Cleaners, guards, laundry personnel, cooks, drivers, and so forth	2,914
Administrator	1,076
Subtotal	3,990
Allied health professional or technician	
Vaccinator	1,954
Laboratory technician	899
Pharmacist	476
Pharmacy technician	244
X-ray technician	134
Technical assistants (X-ray, laboratory, pharmacy, physiotherapy)	107
Dental technician	86
Physiotherapist	31
Orthopedic technician	1
Subtotal	3,932
Outreach worker	
Community midwife	340
Community health worker, male	200
Health inspectors	82
Community health worker, female	53
Sanitarian	7
Community health supervisor	2
Subtotal	684
Manager	
Subtotal	439
Total	17,396

Source: Ministry of Public Health Human Resources Database 2008.
a. A feldsher is an assistant physician trained under the Russian system.

Table F.2   Facilities Other Than Health Centers and Hospitals Not Included in the Facility Inventory, by Province and District

Province/district	Drug clinic	Other[a]	Total
Badakshan			
Fayzabad	1	2	3
Keren-O-Menjan	0	1	1
Subtotal	1	3	4
Baghlan			
Pul-i-Hisar	0	1	1
Subtotal	0	1	1
Balkh			
Mazari Sharif	2	1	3
Subtotal	2	1	3
Bamyan			
Bamyan	1	1	2
Panjab	0	1	1
Waras	0	1	1
Yakawlang	0	1	1
Subtotal	1	4	5
Farah			
Farah	1	2	3
Subtotal	1	2	3
Faryab			
Maymana	1	1	2
Subtotal	1	1	2
Ghazni			
Ghazni	1	2	3
Malestan	0	1	1
Subtotal	1	3	4
Ghor			
Chaghcharan	1	0	1
Lal-o-Sar-i-I Jangal	0	1	1
Subtotal	1	1	2
Hirat			
Hirat	1	0	1
Injil	0	1	1
Subtotal	1	1	2
Jawzjan			
Shibirghan	1	0	1
Subtotal	1	0	1
Kabul			
Kabul	1	6	7
Mir Bacha Kot	0	1	1
Subtotal	1	7	8
Kandahar			
Kandahar	1	4	5
Subtotal	1	4	5

(continued)

Table F.2   *(continued)*

Province/district	Drug clinic	Other[a]	Total
Khost			
Khost (Matun)	0	3	3
Subtotal	0	3	3
Kunar			
Asadabad	0	1	1
Subtotal	0	1	1
Kunduz			
Kunduz	1	3	4
Subtotal	1	3	4
Logar			
Azra	0	1	1
Charkh	0	1	1
Kharwar	0	1	1
Puli Alam	0	1	1
Subtotal	0	4	4
Nangarhar			
Jalalabad	2	1	3
Khogyani	0	1	1
Sherzad	0	1	1
Subtotal	2	3	5
Nimroz			
Zaranj	1	1	2
Subtotal	1	1	2
Panjshir			
Dara	0	2	2
Hisa-I-Awal Panjshir	0	1	1
Uanaba	0	1	1
Subtotal	0	5[b]	5[b]
Parwan			
Salang	0	1	1
Subtotal	0	1	1
Takhar			
Rustaq	0	1	1
Taluqan	0	1	1
Subtotal	0	2	2
Wardak			
Chaki Wardak	0	1	1
Subtotal	0	1	1
Total	16	52	68

Source: Author's compilation, based on documents from the Ministry of Public Health.
Note: None of the districts visited in the provinces of Badghis, Daykundi, Helmand, Kapisa, Laghman, Nuristan, Pakyika, Paktya, Samangan, Sari Pul, Uruzgan, or Zabul had any of these types of facilities.
a. Other facilities include maternal and child health clinics and tuberculosis clinics.
b. Total figure includes a maternal and child health clinic in the Bazarak district.

Table F.3 Surpluses and Deficits in Human Resources, by Job and Province (Badakshan to Kunar)

Type of provider	Badakshan	Badghis	Baghlan	Balkh	Bamyan	Daykundi	Farah	Faryab	Ghazni	Ghor	Helmand	Hirat	Jawzjan	Kabul	Kandahar	Kapisa	Khost	Kunar
Frontline health provider																		
Nurse, male	-36	-39	-35	-40	-3	-102	-22	-28	-173	-83	-35	-17	-58	-802	-42	-35	-33	-19
Physician, female	-30	-12	-16	-7	-3	-47	-14	-15	-32	-32	-16	-13	-26	-21	-17	-12	-14	-8
Nurse, female	-29	-90	-31	-3	28	-43	35	-95	-217	-114	-105	9	-122	-1,107	-70	-69	-60	-67
Midwife	-10	-8	6	-1	7	-5	7	-9	-4	-21	-12	0	25	55	-25	-12	0	-9
Community midwife	-7	-30	-2	-13	-2	-49	0	-27	-101	-55	-41	1	-60	-514	-3	-17	-13	-19
Specialist	-4	-18	-6	-6	3	41	1	-15	12	-13	-17	4	-26	182	-26	-19	-16	-15
Dentist	5	6	-1	8	1	-2	4	-1	-5	-2	-1	0	-3	62	1	1	1	-1
Assistant midwife	9	0	0	8	0	4	2	4	6	0	5	2	0	15	12	0	0	1
Feldsher[a]	17	8	4	17	5	49	11	3	26	58	3	16	13	139	20	6	7	0
Physician, male	35	3	18	31	20	67	46	-8	54	34	8	16	13	-35	9	19	7	3
Subtotal	-50	-180	-63	-6	56	-87	70	-191	-434	-228	-211	18	-244	-2,026	-141	-138	-123	-134

(continued)

Table F.3 (continued)

Type of provider	Badakhshan	Badghis	Baghlan	Balkh	Bamyan	Daykundi	Farah	Faryab	Ghazni	Ghor	Helmand	Hirat	Jawzjan	Kabul	Kandahar	Kapisa	Khost	Kunar
Outreach worker																		
Community health supervisor	−69	−3	−31	−42	0	−4	2	−23	−62	−64	−29	−48	−3	−100	−39	5	−25	1
Community health worker, female	−2	−4	−9	−2	−2	−14	0	4	−31	−3	−7	−7	−4	−2	−9	0	−10	−4
Vaccinator	1	−34	−14	−4	−14	−82	−24	−19	−56	−26	−10	15	−42	1	−1	−26	−6	−6
Community health worker, male	9	−22	−3	2	−7	−79	−18	−1	−17	8	−7	−7	−12	3	−5	−6	−3	0
Subtotal	−61	−63	−57	38	−23	−179	−40	−39	−166	−85	−53	−47	−61	−98	−54	−27	−47	−9
Manager																		
Nursing director/chief nurse	−4	−3	−2	−3	1	−2	−1	−1	−11	−4	−2	−2	2	−26	−4	19	−2	−1
Administrator	−4	−1	−2	−3	0	−3	−1	−1	−11	−4	−2	−2	−1	−26	−4	−1	−2	−1
Hospital director (former doctor)	25	−3	−1	4	0	−5	−1	−1	−5	22	5	6	−2	149	18	−3	4	−1
Medical director	−1	−3	−1	−1	0	−5	−1	−1	−3	−1	−1	−1	−2	−20	−1	−3	−1	−1
Subtotal	16	−10	−6	−3	1	−15	−4	−4	−30	13	0	1	−3	77	9	12	−1	−4

Table F.3 Surpluses and Deficits in Human Resources, by Job and Province (Kunduz to Zabul)

Type of provider	Kunduz	Laghman	Logar	Nangarhar	Nimroz	Nuristan	Paktya	Pakyika	Panjshir	Parwan	Samangan	Sari Pul	Takhar	Uruzgan	Wardak	Zabul	Total
Frontline health provider																	
Nurse, male	-23	-36	-31	-29	-25	-3	-27	-10	-43	-46	-32	-29	-45	-35	-55	-37	-2,110
Physician, female	-16	-5	-17	-11	-12	-13	-13	-3	-16	-11	-7	-165	-8	-14	-30	-16	-604
Nurse, female	19	12	-58	-47	-71	-99	-39	-10	-101	-12	-47	5	-30	-57	-71	22	-2,734
Midwife	4	-15	-4	-2	-13	-16	5	-1	-13	11	5	-2	1	4	-11	3	-60
Community midwife	33	-3	-27	-23	-13	-22	-22	-11	-33	-11	-20	-6	-14	-23	-5	18	-1,134
Specialist	-9	-5	-2	-23	-12	-14	-9	-6	-27	-5	-12	4	3	-17	1	-2	-73
Dentist	2	2	-1	-1	1	-1	1	1	1	6	-1	1	3	0	-2	1	86
Assistant midwife	6	0	2	6	0	0	1	2	1	0	6	0	3	3	2	6	106
Feldsher[a]	1	14	10	18	1	1	13	7	7	3	2	10	6	3	12	17	527
Physician, male	21	60	12	17	2	-2	12	10	21	41	11	44	21	21	17	32	691
Subtotal	38	24	-116	-95	-142	-169	-78	-10	-203	-24	-95	-138	-60	-87	-82	44	-5,305

(continued)

Table F.3 (continued)

Type of provider	Kunduz	Laghman	Logar	Nangarhar	Nimroz	Nuristan	Paktya	Pakyika	Panjshir	Parwan	Samangan	Sari Pul	Takhar	Uruzgan	Wardak	Zabul	Total
Outreach worker																	
Community health supervisor	4	-28	-43	22	-6	-15	-8	-13	-38	8	-20	-1	14	-26	-4	-53	-660
Community health worker, female	-8	-2	-15	-4	0	0	0	-11	-11	2	-6	-7	1	-17	-3	-4	-191
Vaccinator	2	9	-42	2	-9	-22	-1	-4	-21	5	-4	-5	5	-20	-1	29	-424
Community health worker, male	-17	2	-12	-27	0	2	-24	-10	-3	-25	2	-21	-37	-15	-32	6	-376
Subtotal	-19	-19	-112	-7	-15	-35	-33	-38	-73	-10	-28	-34	-17	-78	-40	-22	-1,651
Manager																	
Nursing director/chief nurse	3	-3	-1	0	-1	-2	-1	-1	-4	16	-2	4	13	-2	13	-3	-17
Administrator	-1	-3	-1	-1	-1	-2	-1	-1	-4	-2	-2	-1	-1	-2	-1	-3	-96
Hospital director (former doctor)	-2	5	8	-2	0	-1	-1	1	-2	-4	1	-1	-3	-1	-2	29	236
Medical director	-2	-1	-1	-2	-1	-1	-1	0	-1	-4	-1	-1	-3	-1	-2	-1	-70
Subtotal	-2	-2	5	-5	-3	-6	-4	-1	-11	6	-4	1	6	-6	8	22	53

Source: Author's compilation.

a. A feldsher is an assistant physician trained under the Russian system.

Descriptions of the Four Core Institutional Development Programs of the Health and Nutrition Sector Strategy

Table G.1 Core Institutional Development Programs of the Health and Nutrition Sector Strategy

Program	Objective	Strategies or aims[a]	Subprograms or activities[b]
Policy and Planning Support	Strengthen organizational development and management at central and provincial levels to ensure effective and cost-efficient delivery of quality health care services	• Develop and implement health and nutrition sector policies • Coordinate donors • Establish Ministry of Public Health (MOPH) budget and action plans • Supervise providers of public and private health care services to ensure that they follow government health rules and regulations • Monitor and evaluate quality of health care services • Control norms and standards with regard to health facility infrastructure	• Planning and law enforcement • Monitoring and evaluation and quality assurance • Health Management Information System (HMIS) • Contract Management Unit (coordination body for contracting NGOs and other health care services providers) • Construction • Health care financing (finding ways to support sustainable and accessible health care services)
Human Resource Development and Research Program	Further develop the capacity of health personnel to manage and better deliver quality health care services	• Develop human resources through Public Health Training subprogram • Develop human resources through Ghazanfar Institute of Health Sciences • Conduct research to assess existing health situation, health system performance, and impact through the Public Health Research Subprogram • Serve as center for quality assurance and control for prescribed drugs, foods, safe drinking water, beverages, and cosmetic materials through the Public Health Laboratories Subprogram • Provide quality testing of specimens with public health importance for reference and referral	Current program activities • System of health care registration • Early maintenance of human resources database • Preliminary national testing and certification examination process (in collaboration with Ministry of Education) • Upgraded preservice curriculum for nurses and midwives Planned program activities • Standards for accreditation of training institutes and programs • Standards for accreditation of medical doctors

Subprogram	Strategy	Current and planned activities	Issues
Pharmaceutical Management Support Program	Harmonize the system for procurement of essential medicines for health services facilities	• Procure essential medicines • Manage logistics	• Maintenance of functional drug quality control lab at central level • Distribution of internal productions with assurance of quality • Importation of effective and quality-assured medicine according to national and international standards • Assessment of national drug requirements, in order to avoid shortages at health facility level • Assessment of local use of herbal and traditional medicine and assurance of quality
Administration Program	Develop and maintain equitable, affordable, and sustainable quality support services	• Ensure equitable and affordable support services for lab, blood safety, radiology, pharmaceuticals, equipment, and medical supplies, as well as maintenance of facilities • Manage procurement and logistics using standard international-level procurement, stocking, and logistics systems • Maintain communications and information technology (CIT) • Continue to implement priority reform and restructuring, including the Reform Institutional Management Unit (RIMU) that reports to the Civil Service Commission (CSC) • Enforce public health and private sector laws and regulations	• Fragmentation of procurement units • Fragmentation of financial units • Improvement of intersectoral coordination and communication by units • Improvement of maintenance of equipment and buildings • Lack of CIT, proper database, and absence of a management information system within the administration, notably for procurement, finance, and stock management (data provided are incomplete and unreliable)

Source: Author.

a. Strategies are identified for the Policy and Planning Support Program; project aims are identified for the Human Resource Development and Research Program.

b. Subprograms are identified for the Policy and Planning Support Program; current and planned activities are identified for the Human Resource Development and Research Program.

Figure G.1　Ministry of Public Health Organogram

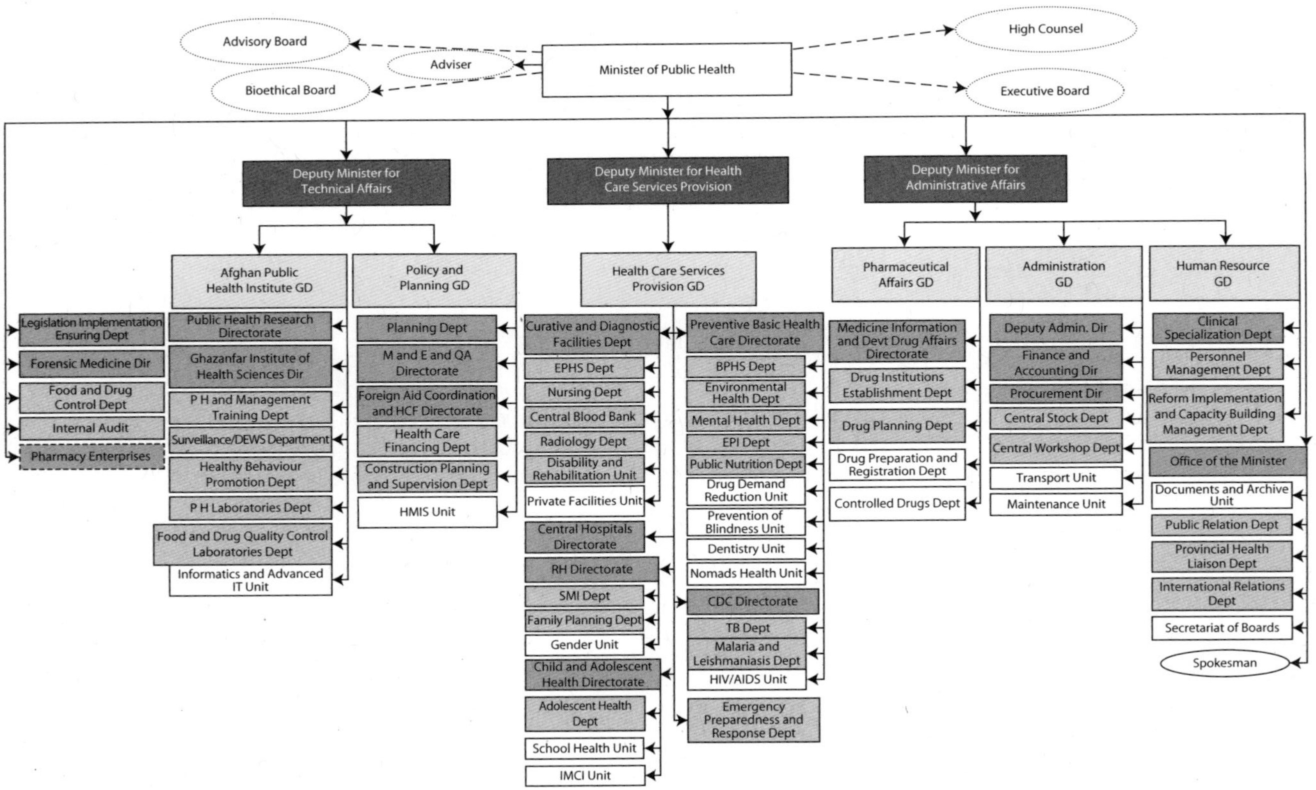

Source: Ministry of Public Health unofficial document (2008).

References

Bartlett, L., S. Mawji, S. Whitehead, C. Crouse, S. Dalil, D. Ionete, P. Salama, and the Afghan Maternal Mortality Study Team. 2005. "Where Giving Birth Is a Forecast of Death: Maternal Mortality in Four Districts of Afghanistan, 1999–2002." *Lancet* 365 (9462): 864–70.

Belay, T. 2009. "Afghanistan: Contracting Management vs. Contracting Service Delivery." Paper presented at Human Development Week, World Bank, Washington, DC, November.

Hendrickson, D., M. Bhatia, M. Knight, and A. Taylor. 2005. "Review of DFID Involvement in Provincial Reconstruction Teams (PRTs) in Afghanistan." CSDG Policy Study 18, Conflict Studies and Development Group, King's College, London.

JHU (Johns Hopkins Bloomberg School of Public Health) and IIHMR (Indian Institute of Health Management Research). 2007. Unpublished results from the Afghanistan Household Survey 2006. Baltimore, MD.

Loevinsohn, B., and A. Harding. 2004. "Contracting for the Delivery of Community Health Services: A Review of Global Experience." Health, Nutrition and Population Discussion Paper, World Bank, Washington, DC.

Loma Linda University. 2008. "Report on Wazir Akbar Khan Hospital." U.S. Agency for International Development project, Kabul.

Ministère des Affaires Etrangères, Government of France. 2007. "Breakdown of Health Expenditure in Countries with High, Intermediate, and Low Income

Levels." Paper presented at the international conference on "Social Health Protection in Developing Countries: Breaking the Vicious Cycle between Disease and Poverty," Paris, March 15–16. http://www.diplomatie.gouv./fr/en/ article_imprim.php3?id_article=8796.

Ministry of Finance, Islamic Republic of Afghanistan. 2007/08. "Annual Budget." Kabul

Ministry of Public Health, Islamic Republic of Afghanistan. 2005. "National Health Policy 2005–2007 and National Health Strategy 2005–2006." Kabul. http://www.moph.gov.af/en/downloads/Policy_2005_2009.pdf

———. 2006. "Afghanistan Household Survey: Estimates of Priority Health Indicators." Kabul.

———. 2007. "Strategic Plan for Monitoring and Evaluation 1386–1390." PowerPoint presentation, November 12.

———. 2008a. "Afghanistan Health Sector Balanced Score Card: National and Provincial Results (2004–2008)." General Directorate of Policy and Planning, Monitoring and Evaluation Unit, Kabul.

———. 2008b. Afghanistan Human Resources Database. Kabul.

———. 2008c. "Health and Nutrition Sector Strategy 1387–1391 (2007/08–2012/13) of the Afghanistan National Development Strategy." Kabul. http://www.moph.gov.af/en/downloads/Strategy_2007_2008_2012_2013.pdf.

MOPH (Ministry of Public Health), JHU (Johns Hopkins Bloomberg School of Public Health), and IIHMR (Indian Institute of Health Management Research). 2007a. "Afghanistan National Health Services Performance Assessment Operations Research Study on Community Health Worker Performance in Afghanistan." Ministry of Public Health, Kabul.

———. 2007b. Drug Quality Assessment Study. Kabul.

MOPH (Ministry of Public Health), UNICEF (United Nations Children's Fund), CDC (Centers for Disease Control), National Institute for Research on Food and Nutrition (Italy), and Tufts University. 2004. "Afghanistan National Nutrition Survey." Centers for Disease Control, Atlanta.

Steinhardt, L. C., H. Waters, K. D. Rao, A. J. Naeem, P. Hansen, and D. H. Peters. 2009. "The Effect of Wealth Status on Care Seeking and Health Expenditures in Afghanistan." Health Policy and Planning 24 (1): 1–17.

Stiglitz, J. 2002. Health and Wealth: Is There a Relationship? World Bank, Development Economics Vice Presidency, Washington, DC.

UNICEF (United Nations Children's Fund). 2004. The State of the World's Children 2004. Girls, Education and Development. New York: UNICEF.

———. 2007. *The State of the World's Children 2007. Women and Children: The Double Dividend of Gender and Equity*. New York: UNICEF.

———. 2009. *The State of the World's Children 2009. Maternal and Newborn Health*. New York: UNICEF.

UNICEF (United Nations Children's Fund), WHO (World Health Organization), World Bank, and UN Population Division. 2007. *Levels and Trends of Child Mortality in 2006: Estimates Developed by the Inter-agency Group for Child Mortality Estimation*. New York: UNICEF.

Vujicic, Marko. 2008. "The Impact of Government Fiscal and Human Resource Management Policies on the Health Workforce in Developing Countries." Draft report, World Bank, Washington, DC.

Waldman, R., L. Strong, and A. Wali. 2006. "Afghanistan's Health System Since 2001: Condition Improved, Prognosis Cautiously Optimistic." AERU Briefing Paper, Afghanistan Evaluation and Research Unit, Kabul.

Weil, D. 2001. "Accounting for the Effect of Health on Economic Growth." Brown University, Department of Economics, Providence, RI.

WHO (World Health Organization). 2006. *The World Health Report 2006: Working Together for Health*. Geneva: World Health Organization.

———. 2007. *World Health Statistics*. Geneva: World Health Organization.

World Bank. 2004. *World Development Indicators 2004*. Washington, DC: World Bank.

———. 2005. "Afghanistan Poverty, Vulnerability, and Social Protection: An Initial Assessment." Human Development Unit, South Asia Region, World Bank, Washington, DC.

Index

Boxes, figures, notes, and tables are indicated by *b*, *f*, *n*, and *t*, respectively.

types of services and providers, 70–73,
71*t*, 72*t*, 171*t*
utilization of public versus private
services, 65, 66*t*
wealth and use of, 67–68
professional councils for health care
professionals, 95, 97*n*4
programs
financing by, 41–44, 42*f*, 43*f*
vertical, 113–14, 128
Provincial Health Coordination Committee
(PHCC) meetings, 129, 140*n*4
Provincial Health Liaison Office, 132, 135
provincial health offices (PHOs), 121*b*,
122–32, 134–40. *See also* Ministry
of Public Health
Provincial Reconstruction Teams,
153, 155*n*1
public health delivery system, 8–9.
See also basic package of
health services; Ministry
of Public Health
public-private partnerships, xxi
public responsiveness and accountability
of MOPH, 121*b*, 130–31, 138

Q

quality of health care
Balanced Score Card. *See* Balanced
Score Card
health care workers, 93–95
private sector, 73–75, 75*t*, 78

R

Red Cross, International Committee of, 37
reproductive health services. *See also*
maternal health
Afghanistan Private Providers Survey
(2008) data, 167*t*, 168*t*
distance from facilities, 27–28, 27*f*, 28*f*
postpartum visitation, 116
private sector, 68–69, 69*t*
trends in coverage of, 21–22, 22*t*
wealth/poverty affecting, 22–25, 24*t*, 25*t*
resource mobilization, 121*b*, 127, 136–37
responsiveness and accountability of
MOPH, 121*b*, 130–31, 138
results-based financing for health
care workers, 108
retrovirus and streptococcal vaccines, 116

rural versus urban areas, financing by, 47*t*
Rwanda, results-based financing for health
care workers in, 108

S

sanitation data, Afghanistan Private
Providers Survey (2008), 167*t*
SCA (Swedish Committee for
Afghanistan), 83
security challenges in Afghanistan, 7–8,
104–5, 105*f*, 106*f*
streptococcal and retrovirus vaccines, 116
subcenters, 101–4, 102*f*, 103*f*
supervisory checklists, 110
Swedish Committee for Afghanistan
(SCA), 83

T

TAG (Technical Advisory Group), 120,
123, 133
Tech-Serve project, 122, 140*n*2
Technical Advisory Group (TAG), 120,
123, 133
technical guidelines and supervision
from MOPH, 121*b*,
131–32, 138
training. *See* education and training
Turkey, bilateral assistance from, 153

U

United Nations, as health sector
donor, 36
United Nations Children's Fund
(UNICEF), 19, 27, 56*n*1,
134, 135, 140*n*4, 152
United Nations Department of Safety
and Security (UNDSS), 7
United Nations Population Fund
(UNFPA), 134, 152
United States Agency for International
Development (USAID), xiii,
1, 10, 11, 12*t*, 33, 45,
100, 132, 154
United States, as health sector
donor, 36, 48, 153
United States Centers for Disease Control
(CDC), 19, 27
urban versus rural areas, financing by, 47*t*
user fees, 40–41
utilization of health care. *See* access
to/utilization of health care

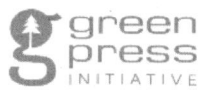